KT-116-658

Medical
Dictionary

BROCKHAMPTON PRESS
LONDON

Revised edition published 1997 by Brockhampton Press,
a member of the Hodder Headline PLC Group.

ISBN 1 86019 018 9

Printed and bound in India

A

abdomen the region of the body which lies below the THORAX, being divided from it by the DIAPHRAGM, and above the PELVIS. The abdominal cavity contains the DIGESTIVE ORGANS (e.g. the STOMACH and INTESTINES), the EXCRETORY ORGANS (BLADDER and KIDNEYS) and, in females, the REPRODUCTIVE ORGANS (WOMB and OVARIES).

ablation the surgical removal (i.e. by cutting) of any part of the body.

abortifacient one of a number of drugs used to bring about an induced ABORTION.

abortion the removal of an embryo or foetus from the womb, either by natural expulsion or by human intervention, before it is considered to be viable at the 24th week of pregnancy. An abortion may be SPONTANE-OUS, and this is commonest during the first three months of pregnancy and is thought to be most often associated with abnormalities in the foetus. Or, an abortion may be INDUCED, when it is also known as THERAPEUTIC, or TER-MINATION OF PREGNANCY, and is carried out for medical or social reasons.

Unless the mother's life is at risk, United Kingdom legislation requires a therapeutic abortion to be carried out before 24 weeks gestation. A THREATENED ABORTION occurs when the foetus is alive but there is bleeding from the UTERUS and/or pain. If the foetus has died the abortion is referred to as INEVITABLE. An INCOM-PLETE ABORTION describes the situation where some of the foetal material is left behind in the uterus.

HABITUAL ABORTION is where a woman loses each foetus in three consecutive pregnancies before the 20th week. The foetus weighs less than 500 grams and an abnormality in the uterus is one of the reasons why this occurs.

ABO system a blood group classification, *see* BLOOD GROUPS.

abrasion a superficial injury caused by the mechanical rubbing off of the skin surface or outer layer of a mucous membrane. Also known as a GRAZE.

abruptio placentae bleeding from the PLACENTA after the 28th week of PREGNANCY which may result in the placenta becoming completely or partially detached from the wall of the UTERUS.

abscess a collection of pus at a localized site anywhere in the body resulting from an infection caused by bacteria. Treatment is by the surgical opening of the abscess and by the administration of ANTIBIOTICS.

abscission the surgical removal of tissue by cutting.

acetylcholine an important organic chemical substance present in the body which is known as a NEURO-TRANSMITTER and is involved in the transmission of electrical impulses along nerves.

achalasia means failure to relax and

usually refers to a condition called achalasia of the cardia. It describes the situation where the muscle fibres surrounding the opening of the OESOPHAGUS (gullet) into the stomach do not relax properly, and hinder the passage of swallowed food.

Achilles tendon this is a large, thick tendon present in the lower leg which attaches the calf muscles to the heel bone enabling this to be moved. It is prone to damage during the playing of energetic sports.

achondroplasia this is the commonest cause of DWARFISM in which the long bones of the limbs are abnormally short. It is inherited as a dominant characteristic in both sexes.

acidosis describes a condition in which the acidity of the blood and body fluids rises to an abnormally high level due to a failure in the mechanisms which regulate the acid/base balance in the body. It is commonly caused by a faulty metabolism of fat, as in DIABETES MELLITUS or during starvation and excessive vomiting.

It may also have a respiratory origin e.g. during drowning when a higher than normal level of carbon dioxide is retained in the body. It also occurs as a result of kidney failure (renal acidosis), when too much sulphuric and phosphoric acids are retained within the body or an excess of bicarbonate is excreted.

acne a disorder of the skin, the commonest of which is *acne vulgaris* in adolescents, characterized by the presence of pustules and blackheads.

SEBACEOUS GLANDS in the skin become overactive (due to hormonal influence) and there is a greater production of SEBUM and proliferation of

bacteria which cause infection. The hair follicles become blocked and pustules form which eventually turn black. The condition usually resolves with time but can be eased with creams and sometimes antibiotics.

Other forms of acne also occur, *see* ROSACEA.

acquired a condition or malady that is not CONGENITAL but arises after birth.

action potential *see* NERVE IMPULSE.

acupuncture a method of Chinese traditional healing involving the insertion of fine needles at various points beneath the skin. The needles are moved by rotation or electric current. The system has been proved to be effective in the relief of symptoms, sometimes being employed as an alternative to ANAESTHESIA.

acute a disease or condition which is short-lived, and which starts rapidly with severe symptoms.

Adam's apple a projection of the thyroid cartilage of the LARYNX which is visible beneath the skin of the throat.

addiction a broadly-used term which describes a state of physical and psychological dependence upon a substance or drug.

Addison's disease a disease caused by the failure of the ADRENAL GLANDS to secrete the adrenocortical hormones, because the adrenal cortex has been damaged. This damage commonly used to be caused by tuberculosis but now, it may more often result from disturbances in the immune system. The symptoms of the disease are wasting, weakness, low blood pressure and dark pigmentation of the skin.

adenitis refers to inflammation of one or more glands.

adenoidectomy the removal, by surgery, of the ADENOIDS.

adenoids a clump of lymphoid tissue situated at the back of the nose (in the nasopharynx). The adenoids may become swollen as a result of persistent throat infections, and obstruct breathing through the nose.

adhesion the joining together of two surfaces which should normally be separate and results from severe inflammation. Bands of fibrous tissue are formed which join the structures together. Adhesions may form within a damaged joint, or following abdominal surgery when they may form between loops of the intestine etc. Adhesions at a joint restrict its movement (ankylosis), and can sometimes be resolved by manipulation. Adhesions within the abdomen or involving the lungs (resulting from PLEURISY), may require surgery

adipose tissue a type of loose, fibrous, connective tissue containing a mass of fat cells. It is a reserve energy store and has an insulating function.

adrenal glands each KIDNEY bears an adrenal gland upon its upper surface. The adrenal glands, also known as suprarenal glands, are important ENDOCRINE organs, producing HORMONES that regulate various body functions. Each adrenal gland has two parts, an outer cortex and an inner medulla which secrete a variety of hormones. Two of the most important ones are ADRENALINE and CORTISONE.

adrenaline a very important hormone produced by the medulla of the adrenal glands which, when released, prepares the body for 'fright, flight or fight' by increasing the depth and rate of respiration, raising the heartbeat rate and improving muscle performance.

It also has an inhibitive effect on the processes of digestion and excretion. It can be used medically in a variety of ways, for instance in the treatment of bronchial asthma where it relaxes the airways. It may be applied to wounds to check bleeding, as it constricts blood vessels in the skin, and also to stimulate the heart when there is cardiac arrest. Adrenaline is also known as epinephrine. *See* ADDISON'S DISEASE.

adrenocorticotrophic hormone (ACTH) is an important substance produced and stored by the anterior PITUITARY GLAND. It regulates the release of corticosteroid hormones from the adrenal glands and is used medically, by injection, to test their function. It is also used in the treatment of asthma and rheumatic disorders.

adult respiratory distress syndrome describes the condition of severe respiratory failure brought about by a number of different disorders. There is a lack of oxygen in the blood, which exhibits itself by imparting a blue tinge to the skin, and rapid breathing and pulse rate. The syndrome may be caused by physical damage to the lungs, by infection or by an adverse reaction following surgery or transfusion. It is often fatal.

aetiology (etiology) the scientific study of the causes of disease.

afterbirth a mass of tissue consisting of the placenta, umbilical cord and membranes, detached and expelled from the womb during the third stage of labour following a birth.

afterpains pains caused by uterine contractions following a birth which help to restore the uterus to its normal size. They may also indicate that a piece of placenta has been retained which the womb is trying to expel.

agoraphobia an abnormal fear of public places or open spaces.

AIDS this refers to *A*cquired *I*mmune *D*eficiency *S*yndrome which was first recognized in Los Angeles in the USA in 1981. The causal agent was identified in 1983 as being the human immunodeficiency virus known as HIV, a ribonucleic acid (RNA) RET-ROVIRUS. The virus has been found in blood, other body fluids, semen and cervical secretions and is mainly transmitted by sexual activity.

The HIV virus affects the T-LYMPHOCYTES of the immune system, and leaves the patient increasingly unable to resist certain infections and tumours which are particularly associated with AIDS. Although they may take a long time to develop, these infections eventually prove to be fatal and at the present time there is no known cure for AIDS.

air embolism a bubble of air in a blood vessel which interferes with the outward flow of blood from the right ventricle of the heart. Air may enter the circulation after an injury, surgery or infusion into a vein. The symptoms are chest pain and breathlessness leading to acute heart failure.

air passages these are all the openings and passages through which air enters and is taken into the lungs. These are the nose, pharynx (throat), larynx, trachea (windpipe) and bronchial tubes. Air entering via this route has dust particles removed, and is warmed and moistened before entering the lungs.

albinism an inherited disorder in which there is a lack of pigmentation in the skin, hair and eyes. The pigment involved is melanin.

albino an individual affected by albinism who typically has pink skin and eyes and white hair. The pink colour is imparted by blood in the blood vessels in the skin which, in a normal person, is masked by the presence of the pigment melanin. Albino people additionally suffer from poor eyesight and have increased sensitivity to sunlight, tending to burn easily.

alimentary canal the whole of the passage along which food is passed starting at the mouth and ending at the anus.

alkalosis an abnormal rise in the alkalinity (a decrease in pH) of the blood and body fluids due to a failure or swamping of the mechanisms which regulate the acid-base balance in the body. It may arise through acid loss following prolonged vomiting, or occur in a patient who has been treated for a gastric ulcer with a large amount of alkalis.

Respiratory alkalosis may arise if breathing is too deep for the amount of physical exertion being undertaken. The symptoms of alkalosis include muscular cramps and fatigue.

allele one of several forms of a GENE at a given place on the CHROMOSOME. They are usually present on different chromosomes and are responsible for certain characteristics of the PHE-NOTYPE. It is the dominance of one allele over another that determines the phenotype of the individual.

allergen any substance, usually a protein, which causes a hypersensitive (allergic) reaction in a person who is exposed to the allergen. There are a great variety of allergens which cause reactions in different tissues and body functions. The respiratory system and skin are often affected.

allergy a state of hypersensitivity in an affected individual to a particular allergen, which produces a characteristic response whenever the person is exposed to the substance. In an unaffected person, antibodies present in the bloodstream destroy their particular antigens (ALLERGENS). However, in an affected individual this reaction causes some cell damage and there is a release of substances such as histamine and bradykin which cause the allergic reaction. Examples of allergies are dermatitis, hay fever, asthma and the severe response known as ANAPHYLAXIS.

alopecia *see* BALDNESS.

alpha fetoprotein a type of protein formed in the liver and gut of the foetus detectable in the amniotic fluid and maternal blood. It is normally present in small amounts in the AMNIOTIC FLUID but when the foetus has a neural tube defect (SPINA BIFIDA and ANENCEPHALY) this level rises higher in the first six months of pregnancy. *See* AMNIOCENTESIS.

alternative medicine the name describes all forms of healing other than western-orientated medical practice and includes acupuncture, homeopathy, osteopathy, naturopathy, faith healing and herbal remedies.

alveolus (*plural* **alveoli**) a small sac or cavity which in numbers forms the alveolar sacs at the end of the BRONCHIOLES in the lungs. Each alveolus is fed by a rich blood supply via capillaries (*see* CAPILLARY) and is

lined with a moist membrane where oxygen and carbon dioxide, the respiratory gases, are exchanged. The alveolar sacs provide an enormous surface area for efficient respiration.

Alzheimer's disease the commonest cause of dementia afflicting those in middle or old age, and a degenerative disease of the cerebral cortex for which there is no cure. Symptoms include progressive loss of memory and speech and paralysis. The cause is not understood but is the subject of ongoing research.

amenorrhoea an absence of MENSTRUATION which is normal before puberty, during PREGNANCY and while breast-feeding is being carried out and following the MENOPAUSE. Primary amenorrhoea describes the situation where the menstrual periods do not begin at puberty. This occurs if there is a chromosome abnormality (such as TURNER'S SYNDROME) or if some reproductive organs are absent. It can also occur where there is a failure or imbalance in the secretion of hormones. In secondary amenorrhoea, the menstrual periods stop when they would normally be expected to be present. There are a variety of causes including hormone deficiency, disorders of the HYPOTHALAMUS, psychological and environmental stresses, during starvation, ANOREXIA nervosa or depression.

amines naturally-occurring compounds found in the body which have an important role in a variety of functions. They are derived from AMINO ACIDS and ammonia and include such substances as ADRENALINE and HISTAMINE.

amino acids the end products of the

digestion of PROTEIN foods and are the building blocks from which all the protein components of the body are built up. They all contain an acidic carboxyl group (-COOH) and an amino group ($-NH_2$) which are both bonded to the same central carbon atom. Some can be manufactured within the body whereas others, the ESSENTIAL AMINO ACIDS, must be derived from protein sources in the diet.

amnesia loss of memory which may be partial or total. *Anterograde* amnesia is the loss of memory of recent events following a trauma of some kind. *Retrograde* amnesia is the inability to remember events that preceded a trauma. Other types of amnesia are *post-traumatic* and *hysterical* and more than one kind may be experienced by an individual.

amniocentesis a procedure carried out to sample the amniotic fluid surrounding a foetus. A fine needle is inserted through the abdominal wall of the mother and the amniotic sac is pierced so that a small quantity of fluid can be drawn off. The amniotic fluid contains ALPHA FETOPROTEIN and cells from the embryo, and various disorders such as DOWN'S SYNDROME and SPINA BIFIDA can be detected. It is usually carried out between the 16th and 20th week of pregnancy if a foetal abnormality is suspected.

amnion a fibrous, tough membranous sac which lines the womb and encloses the foetus floating within it surrounded by amniotic fluid. A 'CAUL' is a piece of the amnion.

amnioscopy the procedure by which an instrument (an endoscope) is inserted either by means of an incision through the mother's abdominal wall or through her cervix, in order to view the foetus. An amnioscope is used if the procedure is carried out abdominally and a fetoscope if through the cervix.

amniotic cavity the cavity, filled with fluid, which is enclosed by the amnion and surrounds the foetus.

amniotic liquid the liquid within the amniotic cavity which is clear and composed mainly of water containing foetal cells, lipids and urine from the foetus. At first it is produced by the amnion but its volume is supplemented by urine from the kidneys of the foetus. It is circulated by being swallowed by the foetus and excreted by the kidneys back into the cavity, and has an important protective function. The amniotic fluid ('waters') is released when the membranes rupture during labour.

amniotomy this refers to the artificial rupture of membranes or ARM which is carried out surgically by means of an instrument called an amnihook. The amnion is ruptured in order to induce the onset of labour.

amphetamines a group of drugs that are chemically similar to adrenaline and have a stimulating effect on the central nervous system. They act on the SYMPATHETIC NERVOUS SYSTEM and produce feelings of mental alertness and wellbeing, eliminating tiredness. They are highly addictive and dangerous and their medical use (mainly in the treatment of hyperkinetic syndrome, a mental disorder in children) is very strictly controlled.

ampicillin a type of semi-synthetic penicillin used to treat various infections and usually given by mouth or by injection.

ampoule a small plastic or glass bubble which is sterile and sealed, usually containing one dose of a drug to be administered by injection.

amputation the surgical removal of any body part but generally refers to a limb.

anabolic (steroids) refers to the effect of enhancing tissue growth by promoting the build-up of protein e.g. to enhance muscle bulk. Anabolic steroids are synthetic male sex hormones (which mimic ANDROGEN), and are used medically to aid weight gain after wasting illnesses and to promote growth in children with certain types of dwarfism. They may also be used in the treatment of osteoporosis. Anabolic steroids should not be taken by healthy people as they have serious side effects especially after prolonged use, and have been misused by athletes.

anaemia a decrease in the ability of the blood to carry oxygen due to a reduction in the number of red blood cells or in the amount of haemoglobin which they contain. Haemoglobin is the pigment within the red blood cells which binds to oxygen. There are a number of different types of anaemia and a variety of reasons for it, and treatment depends upon the underlying cause.

anaesthesia a loss of sensation or feeling in the whole or part of the body, usually relating to the administration of ANAESTHETIC drugs so that surgery can be performed.

anaesthetic a substance which, when administered, produces a loss of sensation in the whole (general anaesthetic) or part (local anaesthetic) of the body. General anaesthetics result

in a loss of consciousness and usually a combination of drugs are used to achieve an optimum effect. These act to depress the activity of the CENTRAL NERVOUS SYSTEM, have an ANALGESIC effect and relax muscles, enabling surgical procedures to be carried out with no awareness on the part of the patient. Local anaesthetics block the transmission of nerve impulses in the area where they are applied so that no pain is felt. Commonly used ones are cocaine and lignocaine and they are used for minor surgical procedures and in dentistry.

anaesthetist a doctor who is medically specialized in the administration of anaesthetics.

analgesia a state of reduced reaction to pain, but without loss of consciousness. It may be due to drugs (*see* ANALGESICS) or it may happen accidentally when nerves are damaged.

analgesics drugs or substances which relieve pain varying in potency from mild, such as paracetamol and aspirin, to very strong e.g. pethidine and morphine.

anaphylaxis a response exhibited by a hypersensitive individual when confronted with a particular ANTIGEN. It results from the release of histamine in body tissues following the antigen-antibody reaction within cells. An allergic reaction is an example of mild anaphylaxis. Anaphylatic shock is a much rarer and more serious condition which can follow the injection of drugs or vaccines, or a bee sting, to which the individual is hypersensitive. Its onset is immediate and results from a widespread release of histamine in the body. The symptoms include severe breathing difficulties, swelling (OEDEMA), a fall in blood pressure, acute URTICARIA and heart failure. Death may follow if the individual is not soon treated with adrenaline by injection.

anaplasia the condition in which cells and tissues become less differentiated and distinctive and revert to a more primitive form. This state is typical in tumours which are malignant and growing very rapidly.

anastomosis in surgery this refers to the artificial joining together of two or more tubes which are normally separate e.g. between parts of the intestine or blood vessels. In anatomy, this is the area of communication between the end branches of adjacent blood vessels.

anatomy the scientific study of the body structure of man and animals.

androgen one of a group of hormones which is responsible for the development of the sex organs and also the secondary sexual characteristics in the male. Androgens are steroid HORMONES and the best known example is TESTOSTERONE. They are mainly secreted by the TESTES in the male but are also produced by the adrenal cortex and by the ovaries of females, in small amounts.

anencephaly a failure in the development of a foetus resulting in the absence of the cerebral hemispheres of the brain and some skull bones. If the pregnancy goes to term the infant dies soon after birth, but spontaneous abortion occurs in about 50% of affected pregnancies. Anencephaly is often associated with SPINA BIFIDA and is the most common developmental defect of the central nervous system. Anencephaly can be de-

tected during the pregnancy by measuring the amount of ALPHA FETOPROTEIN present, *see also* AMNIOCENTESIS.

aneuploidy this describes the condition in which an abnormal number of chromosomes are present in the cells of an affected individual. The number of chromosomes is either more or less than the normal exact multiple of the HAPLOID number (half the full complement) and is characteristic of DOWN'S SYNDROME and TURNER'S SYNDROME, *see* EUPLOID.

aneurysm a balloon-like swelling of the wall of an artery which occurs when it becomes weakened or damaged. There may be a congenital weakness in the muscular wall of the artery involved, as is often the case within the brain. Damage may also be the result of infection, particularly SYPHILIS, or degenerative conditions e.g. ATHEROMA. There is a danger within the brain that an aneurysm may rupture causing a SUBARACHNOID HAEMORRHAGE or cerebral haemorrhage. The surgical treatment of aneurysms has greatly advanced and is very successful in many cases.

angina a suffocating, choking pain, usually used in reference to angina pectoris, which is felt in the chest. The pain is felt or brought on by exercise and relieved by rest, and occurs when the blood supply to the heart muscle is inadequate. During exercise the demand for blood (supplied by the coronary arteries) is increased and if the supply is insufficient, because the arteries are damaged, chest pain results. The coronary arteries may be damaged by ATHEROMA, the most common cause.

Angina pectoris is usually first treated with drugs but if the condition worsens, coronary-artery bypass surgery (ANGIOPLASTY) may need to be performed.

angiocardiography an X-ray examination technique of the activity of the heart involving the injecting of a radio-opaque substance. The X-ray film obtained is called an angiocardiogram.

angiography an examination technique of blood vessels using X-rays, made possible by first injecting a radio-opaque substance. If the blood vessels being examined are arteries it is called ARTERIOGRAPHY and if veins, VENOGRAPHY or phlebography.

angioma a clump of distended blood vessels pushing onto the surface of the brain. It may cause epilepsy and occasionally a vessel may burst to cause a SUBARACHNOID HAEMORRHAGE.

angioplasty a surgical method used to widen or reopen a narrowed or blocked blood vessel or heart valve. A balloon is inserted and then inflated to clear the obstruction.

angitis also known as vasculitis, this describes the condition where there is inflammation of the walls of small blood vessels, usually in patches.

anorexia means a loss of appetite. Anorexia nervosa is a psychological disorder which is commonly associated with young female individuals. The person has a false and distorted image of herself as fat and a fear or phobia relating to obesity, and becomes unable to eat. The person may take laxatives and induce vomiting, as well as starving herself, in order to lose weight. Accompanying symptoms include AMENORRHEA, low blood pressure, ANAEMIA and a risk of sudden death from heart damage.

anoxia the condition when the body tissues do not receive sufficient oxygen. It may be due to high altitudes (and thus lower atmospheric pressure), a lack of red blood cells, or a disease such as PNEUMONIA which limits the amount of oxygen reaching the lung surfaces and therefore reduces that available for transfer to the blood.

antacids substances which neutralize acidity, usually hydrochloric acid in the digestive juices of the stomach. An example is sodium bicarbonate.

antagonistic action an action in which systems or processes act against each other so that the activity of one reduces that of the other. Two muscles may operate in this way, the contraction of one necessitating the relaxation of the other, as in the movement of a limb. In addition, hormones and drugs act antagonistically, the release of one limiting the effect of the other.

antenatal before birth. Pregnant women attend antenatal clinics which monitor the health of both mothers and their unborn babies.

anthrax a serious infectious disease of cattle and sheep which can be transmitted to man and is caused by a bacillus, *B.anthracis*. The spores of the bacillus remain viable for many years and are resistant to destruction. People can be infected by handling contaminated skins, fleeces and bones and the spores may either be inhaled or enter through a cut in the skin. The danger is increased if the infected skins are dry so that spores and dust are inhaled. The disease takes two forms in man, either affecting the lungs (if the spores are inhaled) causing pneumonia (*Woolsorter's disease*), or the skin (if infected through a cut) known as malignant pustule, a severe ulceration.

antibiotic a substance, derived from a microorganism which kills or inhibits the multiplication of other microorganisms, usually bacteria or fungi. Well-known examples are penicillin and streptomycin.

antibodies protein substances of the GLOBULIN type which are produced by the lymphoid tissue and circulate in the blood. They react with their corresponding ANTIGENS and neutralize them, rendering them harmless. Antibodies are produced against a wide variety of antigens and these reactions are responsible for IMMUNITY and ALLERGY.

anticoagulants drugs which delay or tend to prevent blood clotting, examples of which are warfarin and heparin. These are used in the treatment of EMBOLISM and THROMBOSIS to disperse blood clots in vessels.

anticonvulsants drugs which are used to reduce the severity of epileptic fits (convulsions) or to prevent them from occurring.

antidepressants drugs which are administered in order to alleviate depression and its accompanying symptoms.

antidote a substance which counteracts the effect of a particular poison.

antiemetic a drug taken to prevent vomiting, such as are used for travel sickness (*see* MOTION SICKNESS) and VERTIGO.

antigens any substances which cause the formation by the body of ANTIBODIES to neutralize their effect. An-

tigens are often protein substances, regarded as 'foreign' and 'invading' by the body, and elicit the production of antibodies. *See* ALLERGEN, ALLERGY and ANAPHYLAXIS.

antihistamines drugs which counteract the effects of histamine release in the body. They are widely used to treat allergic reactions of various sorts, particularly to relieve skin conditions. Those taken by mouth have a sedative effect and so care must be taken while they are being used.

anti-inflammatory anything which reduces inflammation. Typical anti-inflammatory drugs are the antihistamines, non-steroidal anti-inflammatory drugs (NSAID types used especially in the treatment of rheumatic disease) and glucocorticoids.

antimetabolites a group of drugs used particularly in the treatment of certain cancers which mimic substances (metabolites) present in the cells. The antimetabolites combine with enzymes which would otherwise use the metabolites for cell growth. Hence they reduce the growth of cancer cells but also have attendant side effects which can be severe.

antiperistalsis *see* PERISTALSIS.

antiseptics substances which prevent the growth of disease-causing microorganisms such as bacteria, and are applied to the skin to prevent infection and to cleanse wounds. Examples are iodine and crystal violet.

antiserum a serum that is usually prepared from horses, which contains a high concentration of antibody against a particular antigen. It is injected to give immunity against a particular disease or toxin.

anuria a failure of the kidneys to produce urine which may result from a disorder which causes a prolonged drop in blood pressure. Anuria is typical of increasing URAEMIA and HAEMODIALYSIS may be necessary.

anus the opening of the alimentary canal at the opposite end from the mouth, through which faeces are voided. The anus is at the lower end of the bowel and its opening is controlled by two muscles, the internal and external sphincters.

aorta the major large artery of the body which arises from the left ventricle of the heart and carries blood to all areas. The other arteries of the body are all derived from the aorta.

aortic stenosis a narrowing of the opening of the aortic valve resulting in the obstruction of bloodflow from the left ventricle to the aorta. A common cause of this is calcium deposits formed on the valve associated with ATHEROMA, or damage may have been caused by previous RHEUMATIC FEVER. Also, the condition may arise CONGENITALLY. The effect is that the left ventricle muscle has to work harder in order to try and maintain the blood flow and becomes thicker as a result. The symptoms of aortic stenosis include ANGINA PECTORIS, breathlessness, and the condition is treated surgically by valve replacement.

apgar score a method of assessing the health of an infant immediately after birth carried out at one minute and five minutes after delivery.

aphasia speechlessness caused by disease or injury to the parts of the brain that govern speech-making. Caused by THROMBOSIS, EMBOLISM or HAEMORRHAGE of a blood vessel within the brain as in a STROKE, or by a TUMOUR.

aphonia loss of the voice which may be caused by disease or damage to the LARYNX or mouth or to nerves controlling throat muscles, or may result from HYSTERIA.

aplasia a complete or partial failure in the correct development of an organ or tissue.

apnoea a temporary halt in breathing which may result from a number of different causes. Apnoea is quite common in newborn infants and can be registered by an apnoea monitor which sounds an alarm if the baby ceases to breathe.

apocrine the term for sweat glands that occur in hairy parts of the body. The odours associated with sweating are due to bacterial action on the sweat produced (*see also* PERSPIRATION).

appendicectomy *also* **appendectomy**, this is the surgical operation to remove the vermiform APPENDIX.

appendicitis inflammation of the vermiform APPENDIX which, in its acute form, is the most common abdominal emergency in the western world, usually requiring treatment by APPENDICECTOMY. It is most common in young people during their first 20 years, and the symptoms include abdominal pain which may move about, appetite loss, sickness and diarrhoea. If not treated the appendix can become the site of an ABSCESS, or gangrenous, which eventually may result in PERITONITIS. This arises because infected material spreads from the burst appendix into the peritoneal cavity. Appendicectomy at an early stage is highly successful and normally results in a complete cure.

appendix a blind-ended tube which is

an appendage of various organs within the body. It normally refers to the vermiform appendix which is about 9–10cm long and projects from the CAECUM (a pouch) of the large intestine. It has no known function and can become the site of infection probably as the result of obstruction. *See* APPENDICECTOMY and APPENDICITIS.

areola usually refers to the brown-coloured, pigmented ring around the nipple of the breast.

arrythmia any disturbance in the normal rhythm of heartbeat. The built-in pacemaker of the heart is the sinoatrial node situated in the wall of the right atrium, which itself is regulated by the AUTONOMIC NERVOUS SYSTEM. The electrical impulses produced by the pacemaker control the rate and rhythm of heartbeat. Arrythmias occur when these electrical impulses are disturbed and there are various different types including EXTRASYSTOLES (ectopic beats), ectopic tachycardias, heart block and FIBRILLATION. Most heart diseases cause arrythmias but they may also arise for no obvious cause.

arteriectomy the surgical removal of a part or the whole of an artery.

arteriogram the recording of an arterial pulse which appears as a trace in wave form. It may be recorded on an oscilloscope screen or on a paper strip by various methods.

arteriography the X-ray examination of an artery following the injection of a radio opaque substance.

arteriole a small branch of an artery leading to a capillary.

arterioplasty surgery to reconstruct an artery which is carried out especially in the treatment of ANEURYSMS.

arteriosclerosis a vague term used to describe several degenerative conditions affecting the arteries. *See* ATHEROMA, ATHEROSCLEROSIS.

arteritis inflammation of an artery.

artery a blood vessel which carries blood away from the heart. Oxygenated (bright red) blood is carried by the arteries to all parts of the body. However, the pulmonary arteries carry dark, unoxygenated blood from the heart to the lungs. An artery has thick, elastic walls which are able to expand and contract, and contain smooth muscle fibres. This smooth muscle is under the control of the SYMPATHETIC NERVOUS SYSTEM.

arthritis inflammation of the joints or spine, the symptoms of which are pain and swelling, restriction of movement, redness and warmth of the skin. There are many different causes of arthritis including OSTEOARTHRITIS, RHEUMATOID ARTHRITIS, TUBERCULOSIS and RHEUMATIC FEVER.

arthropathy any joint order or disease.

arthroplasty the operation to repair a diseased joint by constructing a new one, often involving the insertion of artificial materials.

artificial insemination SEMEN collected from a donor is inserted by means of an instrument into the vagina of a woman in the hope that she will conceive. The semen may be from her husband or partner (AIH) or from an anonymous donor (AID) and is introduced near the time of ovulation. Usually AIH is used where the partner is impotent and AID when he is sterile.

artificial respiration an emergency procedure carried out when normal respiration has ceased in order to artificially ventilate the lungs, usually referred to as 'mouth-to-mouth resuscitation.' In hospital where a seriously ill person is unable to breathe unaided, artificial respiration is achieved by means of a machine known as a ventilator.

asbestosis a disease of the lungs caused by the inhalation of asbestos dust. Asbestos dust causes scarring of the lungs. There is a serious risk of MESOTHELIOMA or cancer of the lung.

asphyxia the state of suffocation during which breathing eventually stops and oxygen fails to reach tissues and organs. It occurs as a result of drowning, strangulation and breathing in poisonous fumes.

Also, it can result from obstruction of the air passages either by a foreign body, lodged at the opening (e.g. a piece of food) or swelling due to a wound or infection.

aspiration the process of removing fluid or gases from cavities in the body by means of suction. The instrument used is called an aspirator and various types exist depending upon site of use.

aspirin a type of drug in widespread use which is correctly called acetylsalicylic acid. It is used to relieve mild pain e.g. headache, neuralgia and that associated with rheumatoid arthritis. It is also used to combat fever, and is also helpful in the prevention of CORONARY THROMBOSIS. In susceptible individuals it may cause irritation and bleeding of the stomach lining and is not normally given to children under the age of 12 years. High doses will cause dizziness and possibly mental confusion.

asthma a condition characterized by breathing difficulties caused by narrowing of the airways (bronchi, *see* BRONCHUS) of the lung.

It is a distressing condition with breathlessness and a paroxysmal wheezing cough and the extent to which the bronchi narrow varies considerably. Asthma may occur at any age but usually begins in early childhood, and is a hypersensitive response which can be brought on by exposure to a variety of ALLERGENS, exercise, stress or infections. An asthma sufferer may have other hypersensitive conditions such as eczema and hay fever, and it may be prevalent within a family. It may or may not be possible for a person to avoid the allergen(s) responsible for an asthma attack. Treatment involves the use of drugs to dilate the airways (bronchodilators) and also inhaled corticosteroids.

astigmatism a defect in vision which results in sight being blurred and distorted. It is caused by abnormal curvature of the CORNEA, and possibly the LENS, of the EYE.

ataxia a loss of coordination in the limbs due to a disorder of the CENTRAL NERVOUS SYSTEM. There may be a disease of the sensory nerves (sensory ataxia) or of the CEREBELLUM (cerebellar ataxia). An ataxic person produces clumsy movements and lacks fine control. *See* FRIEDREICH'S ATAXIA and LOCOMOTOR ATAXIA.

atheroma a degenerative condition of the arteries. The inner and middle coats of the arterial walls become scarred and fatty deposits (CHOLESTEROL) are built up at these sites. The blood circulation is impaired and it may lead to such problems as ANGINA pectoris, stroke and heart attack.

atherosclerosis similar to ATHEROMA being a degenerative disease of the arteries associated with fatty deposits on the inner walls leading to reduced blood flow.

athlete's foot a fungal infection of the skin particularly occurring between the toes and often due to RINGWORM.

atrium (*pl.* **atria**) one of the two thin-walled, upper chambers of the heart, which receive blood from major veins. The right atrium receives (deoxygenated) blood from the venae cavae and the left atrium is supplied with (oxygenated) blood from the pulmonary vein. (Atria also refers to various other chambers in the body.)

atrophy wasting of a body part due to lack of use, malnutrition or as a result of ageing. The ovaries of women atrophy after the menopause and muscular atrophy accompanies certain diseases. *See* POLIOMYELITIS.

aural anything relating to the ear.

auricle the external part of the ear of flap known as the pinna. Also, an ear-shaped appendage of the ATRIUM of the heart.

autism a severe mental disorder of childhood in which there is a failure in emotional development and an inability to communicate. There are accompanying behavioural problems and autism may be caused by brain damage and genetic factors. Autistic individuals exhibit stereotyped patterns of behaviour and may or may not be intellectually impaired. They require intensive and prolonged education in order to progress.

autoantibody an antibody produced by the body against one of its own

tissues which is a feature of AUTOIMMUNE DISEASE.

autoimmune disease one of a number of conditions resulting from the production of antibodies by the body which attack its own tissues. For reasons which are not understood the immune system loses the ability to distinguish between 'self' and 'non-self'. Autoimmune disease is currently thought to be the cause of a number of disorders including acquired haemolytic anaemia (*see* HAEMOLYSIS), PERNICIOUS ANAEMIA, RHEUMATOID ARTHRITIS, RHEUMATIC FEVER and DIABETES MELLITUS.

autoclave equipment used to sterilize surgical equipment and dressings, etc. by means of steam at high pressure. It is one of the most important methods of sterilization.

autograft a graft of skin or tissue taken from one part of a person's body and transferred to another region. The graft is 'self' and is not rejected by the body's immune system.

autoimmunity a failure of the immune system where the body develops antibodies that attack components or substances belonging to itself. *See* AUTOANTIBODY, AUTOIMMUNE DISEASE.

autonomic nervous system the part of the nervous system which controls body functions that are not under conscious control, e.g. the heartbeat and other smooth muscles and glands. It is divided into the SYMPATHETIC and PARASYMPATHETIC NERVOUS SYSTEMS.

autopsy or *post mortem*, the examination and dissection of a body after death.

axon *see* NEURON.

B

Babinski reflex a reflex response of the foot (*see* PLANTAR REFLEX). When the sole is stroked the big toe turns up and the others fan out. This is normal for infants up to two years but abnormal thereafter.

bacillus (*plural* bacilli) a term for any bacterium that is rod-shaped. Also a genus of gram-positive (*see* GRAM'S STAIN) bacteria that includes *B. anthracis*, the cause of ANTHRAX.

backbone *see* SPINAL COLUMN.

backache pain in the back which may vary in intensity, sharpness and cause. Much back pain is due to mechanical/structural problems including fractures, muscle strain or pressure on a nerve. Other causes may include tumours, bone disease such as OSTEOPOROSIS, referred pain from an ulcer, or inflammations e.g. SPONDYLITIS.

bacteria (*singular* bacterium) single-celled organisms that underpin all life sustaining processes. GRAM'S STAIN is a test used to distinguish between the two types (Gram positive and Gram negative). They are also identified by shape: spiral, (spirilli), rodlike (bacilli), spherical (cocci), comma-shaped (vibrid) and the spirochaetal that are corkscrew-like. Some are responsible for disease in plants and animals, e.g. tuberculosis, typhoid, syphilis and cholera.

bactericide something that kills bacteria, but used especially when referring to drugs and antiseptics.

bacteriology the study of bacteria.

bacteriophage a virus that attacks a BACTERIUM. The phage replicates in the host which is ultimately destroyed as new phages are released. Each phage is specific to a certain bacterium and uses are found in genetic engineering in cloning and certain manufacturing processes.

baldness the gradual depletion of hair on the head which is to a great extent hereditary. Baldness is a symptom of some diseases, e.g. SYPHILIS, MYXOEDEMA, and anaemia and *alopecia* is a patchy baldness of the scalp that can affect other areas of the body. Baldness is often preceded (for several years) by SEBORRHOEIC ECZEMA which causes hair follicles to lose their capacity to produce hair in the natural cycle of replacement.

ballottement the technique whereby a floating structure in the body can be gently pushed and it then rebounds, e.g. as with a foetus.

bandage a material pad or strip wrapped around a part of the body to hold a dressing in place, immobilize a limb or maintain pressure on a compress.

barbiturate drugs that have anaesthetic, hypnotic or sedative effects. Barbiturates reduce blood pressure and temperature and depress the central nervous system and respiration. TRANQUILLIZERS are replacing barbiturates to lessen drug abuse.

barium sulphate a chemical powder used in X-ray examinations. Due to its opaque (to X-rays) nature, it forms a shadow in whatever cavity it lies. It is used in the examination of the stomach and intestines and can be used to trace a meal through the bowels.

basal ganglion GREY MATTER at the base of the CEREBRUM that is involved in the subconscious control of voluntary movement.

BCG vaccine Bacillus Calmette-Guérin vaccine, named after the two French bacteriologists and first introduced in France in 1908. It is used as a vaccine against TUBERCULOSIS, usually administered intradermally, and complications are rare. A pre-vaccination test is applied to all save the newborn and vaccination is given to those showing a negative result. Vaccination is usually given to: school-children aged 10 to 14; children of Asian origin because tuberculosis has a high incidence in this ethnic group; health workers and others.

bed sores (pressure sores or decubitus ulcer) sore and ulcerated skin caused by constant pressure on an area of the body. Bedridden, particularly unconscious patients, are at risk and their position has to be changed to relieve the prone areas: heels, buttocks, elbows, lower back etc.

Bell's palsy a paralysis of the facial muscles on either or both sides of the face caused by infection/inflammation, when it may be temporary. Permanent paralysis may result from a basal skull fracture, stroke, etc. The paralysis results in an inability to open and close the eye, smile, close the mouth on the side affected.

B endorphin a painkiller released by the PITUITARY in response to pain and stress.

bends (in its complete form also known as compressed air illness or Caisson disease) workers operating in high pressure in diving bells or at depth underwater may suffer if surfacing too rapidly. Pain in the joints (the bends), headache and dizziness (decompression sickness) and paralysis may be caused by the formation of nitrogen bubbles in the blood which then accumulate in different parts of the body. Death may occur.

Benedict's test a test for glucose and reducing sugars. A solution of copper sulphate, sodium carbonate and sodium citrate is added to the sample. The solution is boiled and sugar is indicated by a rust-coloured precipitate. The test is used to detect sugar in urine if DIABETES is suspected.

benign used frequently with reference to tumours, meaning not harmful.

benzhexol (or benzhexol hydrochloride, also trihexyphenidyl hydrochloride) a drug prescribed in the treatment of Parkinson's disease (see PARKINSONISM).

benzocaine used in various forms, a local anaesthetic for relief of painful skin conditions including those within the mouth.

benzodiazepines a group of drugs that act as tranquillizers (e.g. diazepam), hypnotics (flurazepam) and anticonvulsants, depending upon the duration of action.

benzoic acid an antiseptic used to preserve certain pharmaceutical preparations and foodstuffs. It is also used in treating fungal infections of the skin, and urinary tract infections.

benzoin a resin used in the preparation of compounds which are inhaled in the treatment of colds, bronchitis (e.g. Friar's balsam) etc.

benzothiadiazines DIURETIC compounds taken orally, which reduce the reabsorption of chloride and sodium ions in the renal tubules of the KIDNEY. IT lowers of the blood pressure and relieves OEDEMA in heart failure.

benzoyl peroxide a bactericidal agent used as a bleach in the food industry and also as a treatment for ACNE.

beri beri a disease causing inflammation of the nerves and due to a dietary lack of vitamin B₁ (thiamine) which results in fever, paralysis, palpitations and occasionally heart failure.

beta blocker drugs used to treat ANGINA, reduce high blood pressure and manage abnormal heart rhythms. Certain receptors of nerves in the SYMPATHETIC NERVOUS SYSTEM are blocked, reducing heart activity. A notable side effect is constriction of bronchial passages which may adversely affect some patients.

biceps a muscle that is said to have two heads e.g. the biceps of the upper arm (*biceps brachii*) and the biceps on the back of the thigh (*biceps femoris*).

bifurcation the branching of, for example, a blood vessel into two. Also the TRACHEA where it forms two bronchi (*see* BRONCHUS).

biguanides substances, taken orally, that reduce blood sugar level and are used in the treatment of *diabetes mellitus*. The result is that glucose production in the liver is reduced.

bile a viscous, bitter fluid produced by the LIVER and stored in the GALL BLADDER, a small organ near the liver. It is an alkaline solution of bile salts, pigments (*see* BILIRUBIN), some mineral salts and CHOLESTEROL which aids in fat digestion and absorption of nutrients. Discharge of bile into the intestine is increased after food and of the amount secreted each day, most is reabsorbed with the food, passing back into the blood to circulate back to the liver. If the flow of bile into the intestine is restricted, it stays in the blood, resulting in jaundice.

bile duct a duct that carries BILE from the liver. The main duct is the hepatic which joins the cystic duct from the GALL BLADDER to form the common bile duct which drains into the small INTESTINE.

bilirubin one of the two important BILE pigments, formed primarily from the breakdown of HAEMOGLOBIN from red blood cells. Bilirubin is orange-yellow in colour while its oxidized form biliverdin is green. The majority of bile produced daily is eventually excreted and confers colour to the stools.

bioassay the determination of a drug's activity or potency by comparing its effects on a living organism with that of a reference sample of known strength.

biochemistry the study of the chemistry of biological processes and substances in living organisms. Such studies contribute to the overall understanding of cell metabolism, diseases and their effects.

biotin a B-complex vitamin that is synthesized by bacteria in the intestine. A biotin deficiency can occur only if large amounts of egg white are ingested because a constituent, avidin, binds to the biotin.

biopsy an adjunct to diagnosis which involves removing a small sample of living tissue from the body for examination under the microscope. The technique is particularly important in differentiating between benign and malignant tumours. A biopsy can be undertaken with a hollow needle inserted into the relevant organ.

birthmark (*or* **naevus**) an agglomeration of dilated blood vessels creating a malformation of the skin and which is present at birth. These may occur as a large port-wine stain which can now be treated by laser, or a strawberry mark which commonly fades in early life (*see also* MOLE).

bladder a sac of fibrous and muscular tissue that contains secretions. Discharge of the contents is through a narrow opening (*see for example* GALL BLADDER *and* URINARY ORGANS).

blindness being unable to see, a condition which may vary from a total lack of light perception (total blindness) through degrees of visual impairment. The commonest causes of blindness are GLAUCOMA, senile CATARACT, vitamin A deficiency (night blindness) and DIABETES MELLITUS.

blood a suspension of red blood cells (or corpuscles) called erythrocytes, white blood cells (leucocytes) and platelets (small disc-shaped cells involved in BLOOD CLOTting) in a liquid medium, blood PLASMA. The circulation of blood through the body provides a mechanism for transporting substances. Its functions include:

1) carrying oxygenated blood from the heart to all tissues via the arteries while the veins return deoxygenated blood to the heart.

2) carrying essential nutrients, e.g. glucose, fats and amino acids to all parts of the body.

3) removing the waste products of metabolism - ammonia and carbon dioxide, to the liver where urea is formed and then transported by the blood to the kidneys for excretion.

4) carrying important molecules, e.g. hormones, to their target cells.

The red blood cells, produced in the bone marrow, are haemoglobin-containing discs while the white varieties vary in shape and are produced in the marrow and lymphoid tissue. The plasma comprises water, proteins and electrolytes and forms approximately half the blood volume.

blood clot a hard mass of blood platelets, trapped red blood cells and fibrin. After tissue damage, blood vessels in the area are constricted and a plug forms to seal the damaged are. The plug formation is initiated by an ENZYME released by the damaged blood vessels and platelets.

blood count (*or* **complete blood count**, CBC) a count of the numbers of red and white blood cells per unit volume of blood. The count may be performed manually using a microscope, or electronically.

blood groups the division and classification of people into one of four main groups based upon the presence of ANTIGENS on the surface of the red blood cells (corpuscles). The classifying reaction depends upon the SERUM of one person's blood agglutinating (clumping together) red blood cells of someone else. The antigens, known as agglutinogens react with antibodies (agglutinins) in the serum. There are two agglutinogens termed A and B and two agglutinins called anti-A and anti-B. This gives rise to four groups: corpuscles with no agglutinogens, group O; with A; with B and with both A and B (hence blood group AB). The agglutinin groups match those of the agglutinogens, thus a person of blood group B has anti-A serum in their blood. It is vital that blood groups are matched for transfusion because incompatibility will produce blood clotting.

The Rhesus factor is another antigen (named after the Rhesus monkey which has a similar antigen), those with it being Rh-positive and those without Rh-negative. About 85% of people are Rh-positive. If a Rh-negative person receives Rh-positive blood, or if a Rh-positive foetus is exposed to antibodies to the factor in the blood of the Rh-negative mother, then HAEMOLYSIS occurs in the foetus and newborn child. This may cause the stillbirth of the child, or jaundice after birth. Testing of pregnant women is thus essential.

blood poisoning see SEPTICAEMIA.

blood pressure the pressure of the blood on the heart and blood vessels in the system of circulation. Also the pressure that has to be applied to an artery to stop the pulse beyond the pressure point.

Blood pressure peaks at a heart beat (SYSTOLE) and falls in between (DIASTOLE). The systolic pressure in young adults is equivalent to approximately 120mm mercury (and 70mm in diastole). The pressure also depends upon the hardness and thickness of vessel walls and blood pressure tends to increase with age as arteries thicken and harden.

A temporary rise in blood pressure may be precipitated by exposure to cold; a permanent rise by kidney disease and other disorders. A lower blood pressure can be induced by a hot bath or caused by exhaustion.

blood sugar glucose concentration in the blood for which the typical value is 3.5 to 5.5 mmol/l (millimoles per litre). See also HYPOGLYCAEMIA and HYPERGLYCAEMIA.

blood transfusion the replacement of blood lost due to injury, surgery, etc., this may be blood or a component e.g. packed red cells (red blood cells separated from the PLASMA, used to counteract anaemia and restore HAEMOGLOBIN levels). Blood from donors is matched to the recipient for BLOOD GROUP and haemoglobin. Donor blood can be stored for three weeks before use if kept just a few degrees above freezing after which the platelets, leucocytes and some red blood cells become non-viable. Plasma and serum are also transfused.

blood vessel the veins and arteries and their smaller branchings, venules and arterioles, through which blood carried to and from the heart.

blue baby the condition whereby an infant is born with CYANOSIS due to a congenital malformation of the heart. The result is that deoxygenated blood does not go through the lungs to be oxygenated but is pumped around the body. Surgery can usually be performed to correct the condition.

boil (or furuncle) a skin infection in a hair follicle or gland that produces inflammation and pus. The infection is often due to the bacterium *Staphylococcus*. Frequent occurrence of boils may be an indication of DIABETES MELLITUS.

bolus a chewed lump of food ready for swallowing.

bonding the creation of a link between an infant and its parents, particularly the mother. Factors such as eye to eye contact, soothing noises etc. are part of the process.

bone the hard connective tissue that with CARTILAGE forms the skeleton. Bone has a matrix of COLLAGEN fibres with bone salts (crystalline calcium phosphate or hydroxyapatite, in which are the bone cells, OSTEOBLASTS and OSTEOCYTES). The bone cells form the matrix.

There are two types of bone: compact or dense, forming the shafts of long bones and spongy or cancellous which occurs on the inside and at the ends of long bones, and also forms the short bones. Compact bone is a hard tube covered by the periosteum (a membrane) and enclosing the marrow and contains very fine canals (*see* HAVERSIAN CANALS) around which the bone is structured in circular plates (*see also* BONE DISEASES, BONE MARROW).

bone diseases *see* OSTEOMYELITIS, OSTEOCHONDRITIS, OSTEOSARCOMA and ACHONDROPLASIA.

bone marrow a soft tissue found in the spaces of bones. In young animals all bone marrow, the red marrow, produces blood cells. In older animals the marrow in long bones is replaced by yellow marrow which contains a large amount of fat and does not produce blood cells. In mature animals the red marrow occurs in the ribs, sternum, vertebrae and the ends of the long bones (e.g. the femur). The red marrow contains MYELOID tissue with ERYTHROBLASTS from which red blood cells develop. LEUCOCYTES also form from the myeloid tissue and themselves give rise to other cell types.

botulism the most dangerous type of food poisoning, caused by the anaerobic bacterium *Clostridium botulinum*. The bacterium is found in oxygen-free environments, e.g. in contaminated food in bottles or tins. During growth it releases a toxin of which one component attacks the nervous system. It has a very small lethal dose and symptoms commence with a dry mouth, constipation and blurred vision and worsen to muscle weakness. Death is caused by paralysis of the muscles involved in respiration.

bovine spongiform encephalopathy (*or* **BSE**) a disease of cattle that proves fatal and which is similar to scrapies in sheep and CREUTZFELDT-JAKOB DISEASE in humans.

bow legs (or *genu varum*) a deformity in which the legs curve outwards producing a gap between the knees when standing. Small children may exhibit this to some degree but continuance into adult life or its later formation is due to abnormal growth of the EPIPHYSIS.

brachial adjective meaning 'of the upper arm', hence brachial artery etc.

brachycardia slowness of the heartbeat and pulse to below sixty per minute.

bradykinesia the condition in which there is abnormally slow movement of the body and limbs and slowness of speech, as may be caused by PARKINSONISM.

bradykinin a polyPEPTIDE derived from plasma proteins that causes smooth muscle to contract. It is also a powerful dilator of veins and arteries.

brain the part of the CENTRAL NERVOUS SYSTEM contained within the cranium. Vertebrates have a highly complex brain which is connected via the spinal cord to the remainder of the nervous system. The brain interprets information received from sense organs and emits signals to control muscles. The brain comprises distinct areas: the CEREBRUM, CEREBELLUM, PONS, MEDULLA OBLONGATA and mid-brain or MESENCEPHALON. GREY MATTER and WHITE MATTER make up the brain, in different arrangements, and a dense network of blood vessels supplies the grey matter and both blood vessels and nerve cells are supported by a fibrous network, the NEUROGLIA.

The average female brain weighs 1.25kg, and the male 1.4kg and the maximum size occurs around the age of 20, whereupon it decreases gradually. Three membranes (the MENINGES) separate the brain from the skull and between each pair is a fluid-filled space to cushion the brain. There are twelve nerves connected to the brain mainly in the region of the brain stem and four arteries carrying blood to the brain. Two veins drain the central portion and many small veins open into venous SINUSES which connect with the internal jugular vein.

brain diseases many brain diseases are indicated by some impairment of a facility, e.g. a loss of sensation or an alteration in behaviour. *See, amongst others*, APHASIA, CONCUSSION, EPILEPSY, HYDROCEPHALUS *and* MENINGITIS.

brainstem death (*or* **brain death**) a complete and continuous absence of the vital reflexes controlled by centres in the brainstem (breathing, pupillary responses, etc.). Tests are performed by independent doctors, repeated after an interval, before death is formally confirmed. At this point, organs may be removed for transplant providing suitable permission has been obtained.

breast the MAMMARY GLAND that produces milk. Each breast has a number of compartments with lobules surrounded by fatty tissue and muscle fibres. Milk formed in the lobules gathers in branching tubes or ducts that together form lactiferous ducts. Near the nipple the ducts form ampullae (small 'reservoirs') from which the ducts discharge through the nipple.

breast cancer a CARCINOMA or SARCOMA which is the commonest cancer in women. Incidence is low in countries where breast feeding persists and animal fat intake in the diet is low. The first sign may be a lump in the breast or armpit (the latter being due to spread to the lymph nodes). A localized tumour may be removed surgically and in addition, radio, chemo- and hormone therapy can form part of the treatment.

breast screening procedures adopted to detect breast cancer as early as possible. In addition to self-examination, there are many formal programmes of screening.

breathlessness is caused fundamentally by any condition that depletes blood oxygen resulting in excessive and/or laboured breathing to gain more air. The causes are numerous, ranging from lung diseases or conditions (PNEUMONIA, EMPHYSEMA, BRON-

CHITIS) to heart conditions and obesity. In children, narrowing of the air passages is a cause, as is ASTHMA.

breech presentation the position of a baby in the uterus whereby it would be delivered buttocks first instead of the usual head first delivery. The baby, and possibly the mother, may be at risk in such cases.

brittle bone disease see OSTEOGENESIS IMPERFECTA.

bronchiole very fine tubes occurring as branches of the bronchi (see BRONCHUS). The bronchioles end in alveoli (see ALVEOLUS) where carbon dioxide and oxygen are exchanged.

bronchitis occurring in two forms, acute and chronic, bronchitis is the inflammation of the bronchi. Bacteria or viruses cause the acute form which is typified by the symptoms of the common cold initially, but develops with painful coughing, wheezing, throat and chest pains and the production of purulent (pus-containing) mucus. If the infection spreads to the BRONCHIOLES (bronchiolitis) the consequences are even more serious as the body is deprived of oxygen. Antibiotics and EXPECTORANTS can relieve the symptoms.

Chronic bronchitis is identified by an excessive production of mucus and may be due to recurrence of the acute form.

bronchodilator drugs used to relax the SMOOTH MUSCLE of the bronchioles, thus increasing their diameter and the air supply to the lungs. They are used in the treatment of ASTHMA.

bronchus air passages supported by rings of cartilage. Two bronchi branch off from the TRACHEA and these split into further bronchi. The two main bronchi branch to form five lobar bronchi, then twenty segmental bronchi and so on.

brown fat see ADIPOSE TISSUE.

brucellosis a disease of farm animals (pigs, cattle, goats) caused by a species of a gram-negative bacillus, *Brucella* (see GRAM'S STAIN). It may be passed to man through contact with an infected animal or by drinking contaminated, untreated, milk. In cattle the disease causes contagious abortion but in man it is characterized by fever, sweats, joint pains, back and headache.

bruises injuries of, and leakage of blood into, the subcutaneous tissues, but without an open wound. In the simplest case minute vessels rupture and blood occupies the skin in the immediate area. A larger injury may be accompanied by swelling.

bulimia an insatiable craving for food.

bulimia nervosa an overwhelming desire to eat a lot of food followed by misuse of laxatives or induced vomiting to avoid weight gain. Although there is no attempt to hide the condition, it is psychological in origin. There are many similarities with ANOREXIA NERVOSA.

burns burns and scalds show similar symptoms and require similar treatment, the former being caused by dry heat, the latter moist heat. Burns may also be due to electric currents and chemicals. Formerly burns were categorized by degrees (a system developed by Dupuytres, a French surgeon) but are now either superficial, where sufficient tissue remains to ensure skin regrows, or deep where GRAFTing will be necessary.

C

caecum an expanded, blind-ended sac at the start of the large intestine between the small intestine and colon. The small intestine and vermiform appendix open into the caecum.

Caesarian section a surgical operation to deliver a baby by means of an incision through the abdomen and uterus. It is performed when there is a risk to the health of the baby or mother.

calamine zinc carbonate which is a mild astringent and is a component of lotions used to relieve itchy, painful skin conditions such as eczema, urticaria and sunburn.

calciferol a form of VITAMIN D which is manufactured in the skin in the presence of sunlight or derived from certain foods (e.g. liver and fish oils). Its main role is in calcium metabolism enabling calcium to be absorbed from the gut and laid down in bone. A deficiency of vitamin D leads to the bone disease OSTEOLAMACIA and also RICKETS.

calcification the deposition of calcium salts which is normal in the formation of bone but may occur at other sites in the body, *see* OSSIFICATION.

calcium a metallic element which is essential for normal growth and functioning of body processes. It is an important component of bones and teeth and has a role in vital metabolic processes, e.g. muscle contraction, passage of nerve impulses and blood clotting. Its concentration in the blood is regulated by various THYROID HORMONES.

calcium-channel blockers also known as calcium antagonists, these are drugs which inhibit the movement of calcium ions into smooth muscle and cardiac muscle cells. Their effect is to relax the muscle and reduce the strength of contraction and to cause vasodilation. They are used in the treatment of high blood pressure and angina.

callus material which forms around the end of a broken bone containing bone-forming cells, cartilage and connective tissue. Eventually this tissue becomes calcified.

calorie a term applied to a unit of energy which is the heat required to raise the temperature of one gram of water by one degree centigrade.

cancer a widely-used term describing any form of malignant tumour. Characteristically, there is an uncontrolled and abnormal growth of cancer cells which invade surrounding tissues and destroy them. Cancer cells may spread throughout the body via the blood stream or lymphatic system, a process known as METASTASIS, and set up secondary growths elsewhere. There are known to be a number of different causes of cancer including cigarette smoking, radiation, ultraviolet light, some viruses and possibly the presence of cancer GENES (oncogenes).

capillary a fine blood vessel which

communicates with an ARTERIOLE or VENULE. Capillaries form networks in most tissues and have walls which are only one cell thick. There is a constant exchange of substances (oxygen, carbon dioxide, nutrients, etc.) between the capillaries, arterioles and venules supplying the needs of the surrounding tissues.

capsule a sheath of connective tissue or membrane surrounding an organ. The adrenal gland, kidney and spleen are all housed within a capsule. A JOINT capsule is a fibrous tissue sheath surrounding various joints. A capsule is also used to describe a small, gelatinous pouch containing a drug, which can be swallowed.

carbohydrates organic compounds which include sugars and starch and contain carbon, hydrogen and oxygen. They are the most important source of energy available to the body and are an essential part of the diet. They are eventually broken down in the body to the simple sugar, glucose, which can be used by cells in numerous metabolic processes.

carbolic acid phenol derived from coal tar and the forerunner of modern antiseptics. A strong disinfectant, it is used in lotions and ointments such as CALAMINE lotion, but is highly poisonous if ingested.

carbon dioxide also known as carbonic acid, this is a gas formed in the tissues as a result of metabolic processes within the body. Medically, carbon dioxide is used combined with oxygen during anaesthesia. At very low temperatures (-75°C) carbon dioxide forms a snow-like solid known as 'dry ice.' This is used on the skin to freeze a localized area

and also in the treatment of warts.

carbon monoxide (CO) an odourless and colourless gas which is highly dangerous when inhaled, leading to carbon monoxide poisoning. In the blood it has a very great affinity for oxygen and converts haemoglobin into carboxyhaemoglobin. The tissues of the body are quickly deprived of oxygen because there is no free haemoglobin left to pick it up in the lungs. Carbon monoxide is present in coal gas fumes and vehicle exhaust emissions. The symptoms of poisoning include giddiness, flushing of the skin (due to carboxyhaemoglobin in the blood which is bright red), nausea, headache, raised respiratory and pulse rate and eventual coma, respiratory failure and death. An affected person must be taken into the fresh air and given oxygen and artificial respiration if required.

carcinogen any substance which causes damage to tissue cells likely to result in cancer. Various substances are known to be *carcinogenic* including tobacco smoke, asbestos and ionizing radiation.

carcinoma a cancer of the EPITHELIUM, i.e. the tissue that lines the body's internal organs and skin.

cardiac arrest the failure and stopping of the pumping action of the heart. There is a loss of consciousness and breathing and the pulse ceases. Death follows very rapidly unless the heart beat can be restored, and methods of achieving this include external CARDIAC MASSAGE, artificial respiration, DEFIBRILLATION and direct cardiac massage.

cardiac cycle the whole sequence of events which produces a heart beat which normally takes place in less than one second. The atria (*see* ATRIUM) contract together and force the blood into the ventricles (DIASTOLE). These then also contract (SYSTOLE) and blood exits the heart and is pumped around the body. As the ventricles are contracting the atria relax and fill up with blood once again.

cardiac massage a means of restoring the heart beat if this activity has suddenly ceased. Direct cardiac massage, which is only feasible if the person is in hospital, involves massaging the heart by hand through an incision in the chest wall. A method, used in conjunction with artificial respiration, is by rhythmic compression of the chest wall while the person is laid on his or her back. The heel of the hand is placed on the chest in the lower region of the breast bone, and firmly compressed between 60 and 80 times a minute, alternating with mouth-to-mouth resuscitation.

cardiac muscle a muscle unique to the heart, consisting of branching, elongated fibres possessing the ability to contract and relax continuously.

cardiac pacemaker *see* PACEMAKER and SINOATRIAL NODE.

cardiology the area of medicine concerned with the study of the structure, function and diseases of the heart and circulatory system.

cardiomyopathy any disease or disorder of the heart muscle which may arise from a number of different causes including viral infections, congenital abnormalities and chronic alcoholism.

cardiopulmonary bypass an artificial mechanism for maintaining the body's circulation while the heart is intentionally stopped in order to carry out cardiac surgery. A 'heart-lung' machine carries out these functions until surgery is completed.

cardiovascular system the heart and the whole of the circulatory system, which is divided into the *systemic* (arteries and veins of the body), and *pulmonary* (arteries and veins of the lungs). The cardiovascular system is responsible for the transport of oxygen and nutrients to the tissues, and removing waste products and carbon dioxide.

carotid artery one of two large arteries in the neck which branch and provide the blood supply to the head and neck. The paired common carotid arteries arise from the AORTA on the left side of the heart and from the inominate artery on the right. These continue up on either side of the neck and branch into the internal and external carotids.

carotid body a small area of specialized reddish-coloured tissue situated one on either side of the neck where the common carotid artery branches to form the internal and external carotids. It is sensitive to chemical changes in the blood, containing CHEMORECEPTORS which respond to oxygen, carbon dioxide and hydrogen levels. If the oxygen level falls, impulses are transmitted to the respiratory centres in the brain resulting in an increase in the rate of respiration and heart beat.

carpus latin for wrist, consisting of eight small bones which articulate with the ULNA and RADIUS of the forearm on one side and with the *metacarpals* (bones of the hand) on the other.

cartilage a type of firm connective tissue which is pliable and forms part of the skeleton. There are three different kinds, hyaline cartilage, fibro-cartilage and elastic cartilage. *Hyaline* cartilage is found at the joints of movable bones and in the trachea, nose, bronchi and as costal cartilage joining the ribs to the breast bone. *Fibro-cartilage*, which consists of cartilage and connective tissue, is found in the intervertebral discs of the spinal column and in tendons. *Elastic* cartilage is found in the external part of the ear (pinna).

catabolism the biochemical processes within the body (metabolism) are divided into two different sorts - those that build up or produce (synthesize) substances, which is anabolism, and those which break down material (LYSIS) known as catabolism. In catabolism, more complex materials are broken down into simpler ones with a release of energy, as occurs during the digestion of food.

catalepsy a mental disorder in which the person enters a trance-like state. The body becomes rigid like a statue and the limbs, if moved, stay in the position in which they are placed. There is no sense of recognition or sensation and a loss of voluntary control. The vital body functions are shut down to a minimum level necessary for life and, in fact, may be so low as to resemble death. The condition is brought on by severe mental trauma, either as a result of a sudden shock or by a more prolonged depression. It may last for minutes or hours or, rarely, for several days.

cataract a condition in which the lens of the eye becomes opaque, resulting in a blurring of vision. It may arise from a number of different causes including injury to the eye, as a congenital condition (e.g. DOWN'S SYNDROME) or as a result of certain diseases such as DIABETES. However, the commonest cause is advancing age during which changes naturally take place in the lens involving the protein components. This is known as senile cataract. Cataract is treated by surgical removal of the whole or part of the affected lens.

catatonia when a patient becomes statue-like, remaining rigid. It is a symptom of mental disease and often a feature of catatonic SCHIZOPHRENIA. Treatment involves tranquillizers and possibly intravenous barbiturates.

catheter a fine flexible tube which is passed into various organs of the body either for diagnostic purposes or to administer some kind of treatment. One of the commonest kinds are urethral catheters inserted into the bladder to clear an obstruction, draw off urine or wash out this organ.

caul a piece of membrane (part of the amnion) which sometimes partly covers a newborn baby.

cauterize the application of a heated instrument known as a cautery to destroy living tissue or to stop a haemorrhage. It is used in the treatment of warts and other small growths.

cavernous sinus one of a pair of cavities located on either side of the sphenoid bone behind the eye sockets at the base of the skull. Venous blood drains into it from the brain, part of the cheek, eye and nose and leaves through the facial veins and internal jugular.

cell the basic building block of all life

and the smallest structural unit in the body. Human body cells vary in size and function and number several billion. Each cell consists of a cell body surrounded by a membrane. The cell body consists of a substance known as CYTOPLASM containing various organelles, and also a nucleus. The nucleus contains the CHROMOSOMES composed of the genetic material, the DNA. Most human body cells contain 46 chromosomes (23 pairs), half being derived from the individual's father and half from the mother. Cells are able to make exact copies of themselves by a process known as MITOSIS and a full complement of chromosomes is received by each daughter cell. However, the human sex cells (sperm and ova) differ in always containing half the number of chromosomes. At fertilization, a sperm and ovum combine and a complete set of chromosomes is received by the new embryo. *See* MITOSIS and MEIOSIS.

central nervous system the brain and the spinal cord which receives and integrates all the nervous information from the peripheral nervous system.

cephalosporins a group of semi-synthetic antibiotics derived from a mould called *Cephalosporium*. They are effective against a broad spectrum of microorganism and are used to treat a variety of infections. They are sometimes able to destroy organisms which have become resistant to penicillin.

cerebellum the largest part of the hind brain consisting of a pair of joined hemispheres. It has an outer grey cortex which is a much folded layer of grey matter and an inner core of white matter. The cerebellum coor-

dinates the activity of various groups of voluntary muscles and maintains posture and balance.

cerebral cortex the outer layer of grey matter of the cerebral hemispheres of the CEREBRUM. It is highly folded and contains many millions of nerve cells, and makes up about 40% of the brain by weight. The cerebral cortex controls intellectual processes such as thought, perception, memory and intellect, and is also involved in the senses of sight, touch and hearing. It also controls the voluntary movement of muscles and is connected with all the different parts of the body.

cerebral palsy an abnormality of the brain which usually occurs before or during birth. It may arise as a development defect in the foetus due to genetic factors, or by a (viral) infection during pregnancy. A lack of oxygen during a difficult labour or other trauma to the infant can result in cerebral palsy. After birth, the condition can result from haemolytic disease of the newborn, or infection of the brain e.g. MENINGITIS. It can also be caused by cerebral thrombosis or trauma. The condition is characterized by spastic paralysis of the limbs, the severity of which is variable. Also, there may be involuntary writhing movements called athetosis, and balance and posture are also affected. There is often mental subnormality and speech impairment and sometimes EPILEPSY.

cerebrospinal fluid a clear, colourless fluid with a similar composition to LYMPH. It fills the ventricles and cavities in the CENTRAL NERVOUS SYSTEM and bathes all the surfaces of the brain and spinal cord. The brain floats in it and it has a protective function acting as a shock absorber helping to prevent mechanical injury to the central nervous system. The cerebrospinal fluid is secreted by the choroid plexuses in the ventricles of the brain and it contains some white blood cells (but no red), salts, glucose and enzymes. It is reabsorbed by veins back into the blood stream.

cerebrum the largest and most highly developed part of the brain consisting of a pair of cerebral hemispheres divided from each other by a longitudinal fissure. The cerebral hemispheres are covered by the CEREBRAL CORTEX below which lies white matter in which the BASAL GANGLIA are situated. The cerebrum controls complex intellectual activities and also all the voluntary responses of the body.

cervical relating to the neck but often used in connection with the neck of the womb (uterus).

cervical cancer cancer of the neck or cervix of the womb. In the precancerous stage, readily detectable changes occur in the cells lining the surface of the cervix. These can be identified by means of a CERVICAL SMEAR test and, if treated at this stage, the prevention and cure rates of the cancer are very high. The sexual behaviour of a woman influences her risk of contracting cervical cancer. Early sexual intercourse and numerous different partners are now recognized to increase the risk.

cervical smear a simple test, involving scraping off some cells from the cervix and examining them microscopically. The test is carried out every three years to detect early indi-

cations of cancer and is a form of preventative medicine.

cervix a neck-like structure especially the cervix uteri or neck of the womb. It is partly above and partly within the vagina projecting into it and linking it with the cavity of the uterus via the cervical canal.

chemoreceptor cells that detect the presence of specific chemical compounds (present in the nose and taste buds). An electrical impulse is then sent to the brain. *See also* CAROTID BODY.

chemotherapy the treatment of disease by the administration of chemical substances or drugs. It includes the treatment of infectious diseases with antibiotics and other types of drug. Also, the treatment and control of various tropical diseases and, especially in recent years, many different forms of cancer with ANTIMETAB-OLITE drugs.

chest the chest or thorax is the upper part of the body cavity separated from the lower abdomen by the DIA-PHRAGM. The chest cavity is enclosed within the rib cage. The thoracic skeleton consists of the ribs and costal cartilages attached to the sternum (breast bone) at the front. At the back, the ribs join the thoracic vertebrae of the spine. The thorax contains the lungs, heart and oesophagus and above it lies the neck and head.

chicken pox a highly infectious disease which mainly affects children and is caused by the *Varicella zoster* virus. There is an incubation period of two to three weeks and then usually a child becomes slightly feverish and unwell. Within twenty-four hours an itchy rash appears on the skin which consists of fluid-filled blisters. Eventually these form scabs which fall off after about one week. The treatment consists of the application of calamine lotion to reduce the itching, and isolation from other children.

The disease is uncommon in adults as a childhood attack gives lifelong immunity and most children are exposed to chicken pox at some stage. However, the virus may remain within the system and become active later as shingles (HERPES ZOSTER).

chilblain a round, itchy inflammation of the skin which usually occurs on the toes or fingers during cold weather, and is caused by a localized deficiency in the circulation.

chiropody the branch of medicine concerned with the health of the foot including its normal structure and development, diseases and their treatment.

chiropractor a person who practises chiropractic which is a system of manipulation, mainly of the vertebrae of the spine, to relieve stress on nerves which might be causing pain.

chloral hydrate a type of sedative drug which is given mainly to elderly people and children. Within half an hour of being taken by mouth (usually as a syrup), it induces sleep and its effects last for about eight hours. It is useful when used sparingly, but harmful in large doses causing toxic effects and addiction.

chlorhexidine also known as hibitane, chlorhexidine is an antiseptic substance which is used in preparations to cleanse the skin. It is also used in LOZENGES for mild infections of the mouth and throat. Dilute solutions are effective as mouthwash.

chloroform a volatile and colourless liquid which is a compound of carbon, hydrogen and chlorine ($CHCl_3$). It was once widely in use as a general anaesthetic but it affects the rhythm of the heart and also causes liver damage. Hence it is little used today, except in very low concentrations as a preservative and in some LINIMENTS.

choking violent coughing and interference in breathing caused by an obstruction in the airway in the region of the larynx. If the obstruction is large there is a danger of suffocation. If the coughing fails to dislodge the obstruction it is necessary to use other methods to aid a choking person. A child can be held upside down by the legs and struck firmly on the back, as this results in the object being dislodged more easily. With adults it may be necessary to use the HEIMLICH'S MANOEUVRE.

cholera an infection of the small intestine caused by the BACTERIUM *Vibrio cholerae*. It varies in degree from very mild cases to extremely severe illness and death. The disease originated in Asia but spread widely last century when there were great cholera epidemics in Britain and elsewhere. During epidemics of cholera, the death rate is over 50% and these occur in conditions of poor sanitation and overcrowding. The disease is spread through contamination of drinking water by faeces of those affected by the disease, and also by flies landing on infected material and then crawling on food.

Epidemics are rare in conditions of good sanitation but when cholera is detected, extreme attention has to be paid to hygiene including treatment and scrupulous disposal of the body waste of the infected person. The incubation period for cholera is one to five days and then a person suffers from severe vomiting and diarrhoea (known as 'cholera diarrhoea' or 'rice water stools'). This results in severe dehydration and death may follow within 24 hours.

The death rate is low (5%) in those given proper and prompt treatment but the risk is greater in children and the elderly. Vaccination against cholera can be given but it is only effective for about 6 months.

cholesterol a fatty insoluble molecule (sterol), which is widely found in the body and is synthesized from saturated fatty acids in the liver. Cholesterol is an important substance in the body being a component of cell membranes and a precursor in the production of steroid hormones (sex hormones) and bile salts. An elevated level of blood cholesterol is associated with ATHEROMA which may result in high blood pressure and coronary thrombosis, and this is seen in the disease, DIABETES MELLITUS. It is generally recommended that people should reduce their consumption of saturated fat and look for alternatives in the form of unsaturated fats which are found in vegetable oils.

choluria bile in the urine which occurs when there is an elevated level of bile in the blood. This may result from the condition known as obstructive JAUNDICE when the bile ducts become obstructed so that bile manufactured in the liver fails to reach the intestine. The urine is dark coloured and contains bile salts.

chorea a disorder of the nervous system characterized by the involuntary, jerky movements of the muscles mainly of the face, shoulders and hips. *Sydenham's chorea* or *St. Vitus' Dance* is a disease that mainly affects children and is associated with acute rheumatism. About one third of affected children develop rheumatism elsewhere in the body, often involving the heart, and the disease is more common in girls than in boys. If the heart is affected there may be problems in later life but treatment consists of rest and the giving of mild sedatives. The condition usually recovers over a period of a few months. *Huntington's chorea* is an inherited condition which does not appear until after the age of 40 and is accompanied by dementia. *Senile chorea* afflicts some elderly people but there is no dementia. *See also* RHEUMATIC FEVER.

chorionic gonadotrophic hormone a hormone produced during pregnancy by the placenta, large amounts of which are present in the urine of a pregnant woman. The presence of this hormone is the basis of most pregnancy tests. Also known as human chorionic gonadotrophin (HCG), it is given by injection to treat cases of delayed puberty and, with another hormone called follicle stimulating hormone, women who are sterile due to a failure in ovulation. It is also used to treat premenstrual tension.

choroid plexus an extensive network of blood vessels present in the ventricles of the brain and responsible for the production of the CEREBROSPINAL FLUID.

chromosomes the rodlike structures

present in the nucleus of every body cell which carry the genetic information or genes. Each human body cell contains twenty-three pairs of chromosomes (apart from the sperm and ova), half derived from the mother and half from the father. Each chromosome consists of a coiled double filament (double helix) of DNA with genes carrying the genetic information arranged linearly along its length. The genes determine all the characteristics of each individual. Twenty-two of the pairs of chromosomes are the same in males and females. The twenty-third pair are the sex chromosomes and males have one X and one Y whereas females have two X chromosomes. *See* CELL and SEX-LINKED INHERITANCE.

chyme the partly digested food which passes from the stomach into the intestine. It is produced by the mechanical movements of the stomach and the acid secretions present in the gastric juice.

cilia fine hair-like projections found lining the epithelium of the upper respiratory tract. These beat and help to maintain the flow of air and remove and trap particles of dust.

circulation of the blood the basic circulation is as follows: all the blood from the body returns to the heart via the veins, eventually entering the right atrium through the inferior and superior venae cavae. This contracts and forces the blood into the right ventricle and from there is driven to the lungs via the pulmonary artery. In the lungs, oxygen is taken up and carbon dioxide is released and the blood then passes into the pulmonary veins and is returned to the left

atrium of the heart. Blood is forced from the left atrium into the left ventricle and from there into the aorta. The aorta branches giving off the various arteries which carry the blood to all the different parts of the body. The blood eventually enters the fine network of arterioles and capillaries and supplies all the tissues and organs with oxygen and nutrients. It passes into the venules and veins, eventually returning to the right atrium through the vena cavae to complete the cycle.

circumcision a surgical removal of the FORESKIN (or prepuce) of the penis in males and part or all of the external genitalia (CLITORIS, labia minora, labia majora) in females. In females and usually in males, the procedure is carried out for religious reasons. Male circumcision may be required in the medical conditions known as PHIMOSIS and PARAPHIMOSIS. Female circumcision is damaging and not beneficial to a woman's health.

cirrhosis a disease of the liver in which fibrous tissue resembling scar tissue is produced as a result of damage and death to the cells. The liver becomes yellow-coloured and nodular in appearance, and there are various types of the disease including alcoholic cirrhosis and postnecrotic cirrhosis caused by viral hepatitis. The cause of the cirrhosis is not always found (cryptogenic cirrhosis) but the progress of the condition can be halted if this can be identified and removed. This particularly is applicable in alcoholic cirrhosis where the consumption of alcohol has to cease.

clavicle the collar bone forming a part of the shoulder girdle of the skeleton. It is the most commonly fractured bone in the body.

cleft palate a developmental defect in which a fissure is left in the midline of the palate as the two sides fail to fuse. It may also involve the lip (HARELIP) and the condition is corrected by surgery.

clitoris a small organ present in females, situated where the labial folds meet below the pubic bone. It contains erectile tissue which enlarges and hardens with sexual stimulation.

clone a group of cells that are derived from one cell (by asexual division) and are genetically identical.

clostridium a group of bacteria which are present in the intestine of man and animals. Some species are responsible for diseases such as botulism, tetanus and gas GANGRENE.

clot the term applied to a semisolid lump of blood or other fluid in the body. A blood clot consists of a fine network of FIBRIN in which blood corpuscles are caught, *see* COAGULATION.

coagulation (of the blood) the natural process in which blood is converted from a liquid to a semisolid state to arrest bleeding (haemorrhage). A substance known as prothrombin and calcium are normally present in the blood, and the enzyme thromboplastin is present in the platelets (*see* BLOOD). When bleeding occurs, thromboplastin is released and prothrombin and calcium are converted by the enzyme into THROMBIN. A soluble protein called fibrinogen is always present in the blood and is converted by thrombin into FIBRIN which is the final stage in the coagulation process. A fibrous meshwork or clot is produced consisting of fibrin and

blood cells which seals off the damaged blood vessel. In normal conditions, thromboplastin is not released and so a clot cannot form. The coagulation or clotting time is the time taken for blood to clot and is normally between three to eight minutes.

coagulation factors these are substances present in plasma which are involved in the process of blood coagulation. They are designated by a set of Roman numerals, e.g. Factor VIII, and lack of any of them means that the blood is unable to clot. *See* HAEMOPHILIA.

cocaine an alkaloid substance derived from the leaves of the coca plant which is used as a local anaesthetic in nose, throat, ear and eye surgery. It has a stimulating effect on the central nervous system when absorbed, in which fatigue and breathlessness (caused by exertion) disappear. However, it is highly addictive and damaging to the body if it is used often and hence it is very strictly controlled. It is also one of the drugs given for pain relief in cases of terminal cancer.

coccyx the end of the backbone, which consists of four fused and reduced vertebrae which correspond to the tail of other mammals. The coccyx is surrounded by muscle and joins with the SACRUM, a further group of fused vertebrae which is part of the PELVIS.

cochlea a spiral-shaped organ resembling a snail shell forming a part of the inner ear and concerned with hearing. It consists of three fluid-filled canals with receptors which detect pressure changes caused by sound waves. Nerve impulses are sent to the brain where the information is received and decoded.

codeine a substance derived from morphine which is used for pain relief and to suppress a cough.

cod liver oil oil derived from the pressed fresh liver of cod which is a rich source of vitamins D and A, and is used as a dietary supplement.

coeliac disease also known as gluten enteropathy, this is a wasting disease of childhood in which the intestines are unable to absorb fat. The intestinal lining is damaged due to a sensitivity to the protein gluten which is found in wheat and rye flour. An excess of fat is excreted and the child fails to grow and thrive. Successful treatment is by adhering strictly to a gluten-free diet throughout life.

cold (common cold) widespread and mild infection of the upper respiratory tract caused by a virus. There is inflammation of the mucous membranes and symptoms include feverishness, coughing, sneezing, runny nose, sore throat, headache and sometimes face ache due to catarrh in the SINUSES. The disease is spread by coughing and sneezing and treatment is by means of bed rest and the taking of mild ANALGESICS.

cold sore *see* HERPES SIMPLEX.

colectomy surgical removal of the colon.

colic spasmodic, severe abdominal pain which occurs in waves with brief interludes in between. Intestinal colic is usually the result of the presence of some indigestible food which causes the contraction of the intestinal muscles. Infantile colic, common in young babies, is due to wind associated with feeding. An attack of colic is generally not serious but can result in a twisting of the bowel which must receive immediate medical attention. Colic-type pain may also be caused by an obstruction in the bowel such as a tumour which again requires early medical treatment.

colitis inflammation of the colon, the symptoms of which include abdominal pain and diarrhoea, sometimes bloodstained. *Ulcerative colitis* tends to affect young adults and tends to occur periodically over a number of years. There is abdominal discomfort, fever, frequent watery diarrhoea containing mucus and blood, and anaemia. The condition can be fatal but usually there is a gradual recovery. Treatment is by means of bed rest, drug treatment with corticosteroids and iron supplements, and a bland, low roughage diet. Colitis may be due to infections caused by the organism *Entamoeba histolytica* (amoebic colitis) and by bacteria (infective colitis). It may also occur in CROHN'S DISEASE.

collagen a protein substance that is widely found in the body in connective tissue, tendons, skin, cartilage, bone and ligaments. It plays a major part in conferring tensile strength to various body structures.

collar bone *see* CLAVICLE.

colon the main part of the large intestine which removes water and salts from the undigested food passed into it from the small intestine. When water has been extracted the remains of the food (faeces) are passed on to the rectum.

colostomy a surgical operation to produce an artificial opening of the colon through the abdominal wall. The colostomy may only be temporary, as part of the management of a patient's condition, e.g. to treat an obstruction in the colon or rectum. However, if the rectum or part of the colon have been removed because of cancer the colostomy is permanent and functions as the anus.

colostrum the first fluid produced by the mammary glands of the breasts after birth. It is a fairly clear fluid containing antibodies, serum and white blood cells and is produced during the first two or three days prior to the production of milk.

colour blindness a general term for a number of conditions in which there is a failure to distinguish certain colours. It is more prevalent in males than in females and is usually inherited. The most common form is Daltonism in which reds and greens are confused. This is a sex-linked disorder, the recessive gene responsible being carried on the X chromosome and hence more likely to be present in males. The cause of colour blindness is thought to be due to a failure in the operation of the CONES, the light-sensitive cells in the RETINA of the eye which detect colours.

coma a state of deep unconsciousness from which a person cannot be roused. There may be an absence of pupillary and corneal reflexes and no movements of withdrawal when painful stimuli are applied. It may be accompanied by deep, noisy breathing and strong heart action and is caused by a number of different conditions. These include apoplexy, high fever, brain injury, diabetes mellitus, carbon monoxide poison-

ing and drug overdose. A comatose person may eventually die but can recover depending upon the nature of the coma and its cause.

comminuted fracture a serious injury to a bone in which more than one break occurs accompanied by splintering and damage to the surrounding tissues. It usually results from a crushing force, with damage to nerves, muscles and blood vessels, and the bone is difficult to set.

commissure a joining or connection of two similar structure on either side of a mid-line. It is usually applied to bundles of nerve fibres connecting the right and left side of the brain and spinal cord.

compress a pad soaked in hot or cold water, wrung out and applied to an inflamed or painful part of the body. A hot compress is called a fomentation.

computerized tomography a diagnostic technique in radiology whereby 'slices' of the body are recorded using a special X-ray scanner known as a CT scanner. The information is integrated by computer to give an image in cross-section of the tissue under investigation. The technique is used for investigations of the brain, for example if a tumour, haematoma or abscess is present. Whole body scans may be required for a number of conditions, but are particularly useful when malignancy is present, supplying information about the position and outline of a tumour and the extent of spread of cancer.

concretions hard, stony masses of various sizes formed within the body. Also known as calculi (single, *calculus*).

concussion a loss of consciousness

caused by a blow to the head. The sudden knock to the head causes a compression wave which momentarily interrupts the blood supply to the brain. The unconsciousness may last for seconds or hours and when the person comes round there may be some headache and irritability which can last for some time. A mild case of concussion may not involve complete loss of consciousness but be marked by giddiness, confusion and headache. In all cases, the person needs to rest and remain under observation.

condyle a rounded knob that is found at the ends of some bones e.g. on the femur and humerus and articulates with an adjacent bone.

cone a type of photoreceptor (light-sensitive cell) found in the RETINA of the eye which detects colour. Cones contain the pigment retinene and the protein opsin and there are three different types which react to light of differing wavelengths, (blue, green and red).

congenital diseases or conditions that are present at birth.

conjunctivitis inflammation of the mucous membrane (conjunctiva) that lines the inside of the eyelid and covers the front of the eye. The eyes become pink and watery and the condition is usually caused by an infection which may be bacterial, viral or the microorganism *Chlamydia* may be responsible.

connective tissue supporting or packing tissue within the body which holds or separates other tissues and organs. It consists of a ground material composed of substances called mucopolysaccharides. In this, certain fibres such as yellow elastic, white collagenous and reticular fibres are embedded along with a variety of other cells, e.g. MAST CELLS, MACROPHAGES, fibroblasts and fat cells. The constituents vary in proportions in different kinds of connective tissue to produce a number of distinct types. Examples are adipose (fatty) tissue, cartilage, bone, tends and ligaments.

constipation the condition in which the bowels are opened too infrequently and the faeces become dry, hard and difficult and painful to pass. The frequency of normal bowel opening varies between people but when constipation becomes a problem, it is usually a result of inattention to this habit or to the diet. Constipation is also a symptom of the more serious condition of blockage of the bowel (by a tumour), but this is less common.

contraception prevention of conception. Pregnancy can be prevented by *barrier methods* in which there is a physical barrier to prevent the sperm from entering the cervix: the condom (sheath) and diaphragm (cap). As well as being a contraceptive the sheath reduces the risk of either partner contracting a sexually transmitted disease including HIV infection. Non-barrier methods include the IN-TRAUTERINE CONTRACEPTIVE DEVICE (coil) and oral contraceptives (the Pill) which are hormonal preparations. Depot preparations are also hormonal drugs given by injection, in subcutaneous implants and released from intravaginal rings.

Sterilization of either a man or woman provides a means of permanent contraception. It is also possible to give a high dose of oral contraceptives within 72 hours of unprotected intercourse, but this is usually regarded as an emergency method. The rhythm method of contraception involves restricting sexual intercourse to certain days of a woman's monthly cycle when conception is least likely to occur.

controlled drugs those drugs which, in the United Kingdom, are subject to the restrictions of the Misuse of Drugs Act 1971. They are classified into three categories: Class A includes LSD, morphine, cocaine and pethidine. Class B includes cannabis, amphetamines and barbiturates and Class C comprises amphetamine-related drugs and some others.

convulsions also known as fits, these are involuntary, alternate, rapid, muscular contractions and relaxations throwing the body and limbs into contortions. They are caused by a disturbance of brain function and in adults usually result from epilepsy. In babies and young children they occur quite commonly but are generally not serious. Causes include a high fever due to infection, brain diseases such as meningitis and breath-holding, which is quite common in infants and very young children. Unless they are caused by the presence of disease or infection which requires to be treated, they are rarely life-threatening.

cornea the outermost, exposed layer of the EYE which is transparent and lies over the iris and lens. It refracts light entering the eye, directing the rays to the lens and thus acting as a coarse focus. It is a layer of connective tissue which has no blood supply of its own but is supplied with nutrients from fluid within the eye (the aqueous humour). It is highly sensitive to pain and presence or absence of response if the cornea is touched is used as an indicator of a person's condition, for example in a comatose patient.

corneal graft also known as keratoplasty, is a surgical procedure to replace a damaged or diseased cornea with one from a donor. Sometimes only the outer layers of the cornea are replaced (lamellar keratoplasty) or the whole structure may be involved (penetrating keratoplasty).

corn (and bunion) a small, localized portion of hardened, thickened skin occurring on or between the toes which is cone-shaped. The point of the cone, known as 'the eye' points inwards and causes pain. It is caused by pressure from poorly-fitting shoes. A bunion is found over the joint at the base of the largest toe and is also caused by tightfitting footwear. With a bunion, the joint between the toe and the first metatarsal bone becomes swollen and forms a lump beneath the thickened skin, due to bending caused by the shoe. A hammer toe is similar but involves the second toe which becomes bent at the joint to resemble a hammer because shoes or boots are too tight or pointed.

coronary angioplasty *see* ANGIOPLASTY.

coronary arteries the arteries that supply blood to the heart and which arise from the AORTA.

coronary artery disease any abnormal condition that affects the arteries of the heart. The commonest disease is coronary ATHEROSCLEROSIS. ANGINA is a common symptom.

coronary bypass graft a surgical operation which is carried out when one or more of the coronary arteries have become narrowed by disease (ATHEROMA). A section of vein from a leg is grafted in to bypass the obstruction and this major operation is usually successful and greatly improves a person's quality of life.

coronary thrombosis a sudden blockage of one of the coronary arteries by a blood clot or thrombus which interrupts the blood supply to the heart. The victim collapses with severe and agonizing chest pain often accompanied by vomiting and nausea. The skin becomes pale and clammy, the temperature rises and there is difficulty in breathing. Coronary thrombosis generally results from ATHEROMA, and the part of the heart muscle which has its blood supply disrupted dies, a condition known as MYOCARDIAL INFARCTION. Specialist care in a coronary care unit is usually required to deal with ARRHYTHMIA, heart failure and CARDIAC ARREST which are the potentially fatal results of coronary thrombosis.

corpus luteum the tissue that forms within the ovary after a Graafian follicle (the structure which contains the egg) ruptures and releases an ovum at the time of OVULATION. It consists of a mass of cells containing yellow, fatty substances, and secretes the hormone PROGESTERONE which prepares the womb to receive a fertilized egg. If the egg is not fertilized and no implantation of an embryo takes place, the corpus luteum degenerates. However, if a pregnancy ensues, the corpus luteum expands and secretes progesterone until this function is taken over by the placenta at the fourth month.

cortex the outer part of an organ situated beneath its enclosing capsules or outer membrane. Examples are the adrenal cortex of the adrenal glands, renal cortex of the kidneys and cerebral cortex of the brain.

corticosteroids any steroid hormone manufactured by the adrenal cortex of which there are two main types. *Glucocorticosteroids* such as cortisol and cortisone are required by the body mainly for glucose metabolism and for responding to stress. *Mineralocorticosteroids*, e.g. aldosterone regulate the salt and water balance. Both groups are manufactured synthetically and used in the treatment of various disorders.

cortisone a glucocorticosteroid hormone produced by the adrenal cortex. It is used medically to treat deficiency of corticosteroid hormones. Deficiency occurs in ADDISON'S DISEASE and if the adrenal glands have had to be surgically removed for some reason. Its use is restricted because it causes severe side effects including damage to the muscle, bone, eye changes, stomach ulcers and bleeding as well as nervous and hormonal disturbances.

costal cartilage a type of cartilage connecting a rib to the sternum (breastbone).

cot death *see* SUDDEN INFANT DEATH SYNDROME.

cradlecap a form of seborrhoea or dermatitis of the scalp which affects young babies and responds to an ointment containing white soft paraffin, salicylic acid and sulphur.

cramp prolonged and painful spasmodic muscular contraction which often occurs in the limbs but can affect certain internal organs (*see* COLIC and GASTRALGIA). Cramp may result from a salt imbalance as in heat cramp. Working in high temperatures causes excessive sweating and consequent loss of salt. It can be corrected and prevented by an increase of the salt intake. Occupational cramp results from continual repetitive use of particular muscles. Night cramp occurs during sleep and is especially common among elderly people, diabetics and pregnant women. The cause is not known.

cranial nerves twelve pairs of nerves which arise directly from the brain each with dorsal and ventral branches known as *roots*. Each root remains separate and is assigned a roman numeral as well as a name. Some cranial nerves are mainly sensory while others are largely motor and they leave the skull through separate apertures. The cranial and spinal nerves are an important part of the *peripheral nervous system* which comprises all parts lying outside the brain and spinal cord.

cranium the part of the skull that encloses the brain, formed from eight fused and flattened bones that are joined by immovable suture JOINTS.

crepitus the grating sound heard when the ends of fractured bones rub together, and also from arthritic joints. It also occurs in *chondromalacia patellae* which is a roughening of the inner surface of the kneecap which produces the grating sound and pain. Crepitus also denotes the sound heard by means of a STETHO-SCOPE from an inflamed lung when there is fluid in the alveoli.

cretinism a syndrome caused by lack of thyroid hormone which is present before birth and is also called *congenital hyperthyroidism*. It is characterized by dwarfism, mental retardation and coarseness of skin and hair. Early diagnosis and treatment with thyroid extract (thyroxine) is vital as this greatly improves a child's intellectual and other abilities. In the UK, blood serum from newborn babies is tested for thyroxine level in order to detect this condition.

Creutzfeldt-Jakob disease also known as spongiform encephalopathy, this is a fatal disease of the brain thought to be caused by a SLOW VIRUS. There is a spongy degeneration of the brain and rapid progressive dementia. The disease usually strikes in middle and early old age and is usually fatal within a year. Similar diseases in animals are bovine spongiform encephalopathy (BSE) in cattle and scrapie in sheep which, it is alleged by some scientists, may be transmittable to man. Recently there has been alarm that some adults treated in childhood for dwarfism with extracts of pituitary glands obtained from corpses, may be at risk of contracting Creutzfeldt-Jakob disease. It is alleged that some of the pituitary glands obtained may have been infected with the virus and that the disease has been passed on and has already caused some deaths.

croup a group of diseases characterized by a swelling, partial obstruction and inflammation of the entrance to the larynx, occurring in young children. The breathing is harsh and strained producing a typical crowing sound, accompanied by coughing and feverishness. Diphtheria used to be a common cause of croup but it now usually results from a viral infection of the respiratory tract (LARYNGO-TRACHEO BRONCHITIS). The condition is relieved by inhaling steam (a soothing preparation such as tincture of benzoin is sometimes added to the hot water) and also by mild sedatives and/or pain killers. Rarely, the obstruction completely blocks the larynx in which case emergency TRACHEOSTOMY or nasotracheal INTUBATION may be required. Usually, the symptoms of croup subside, but the child may have a tendency towards future attacks.

cryosurgery the use of extreme cold to perform surgical procedures, usually on localized areas to remove unwanted tissue. The advantages are that there is little or no bleeding or sensation of pain, and scarring is very much reduced. An instrument called a cryoprobe is used, the fine tip of which is cooled by means of a coolant substance contained within the probe. The coolants used are carbon dioxide ad nitrous oxide gas and liquid nitrogen. Cryosurgery is used for the removal of cataracts, warts and to destroy some bone tumours.

culture a population of bacteria viruses other microorganisms, or cells grown in the laboratory on a nutrient base known as a *culture medium*.

Cushing's syndrome a metabolic disorder which results from excessive amounts of CORTICOSTEROIDS in the body due to an inability to regulate cortisol or adrenocorticotropic hormone (ACTH). The commonest cause is a tumour of the PITUITARY GLAND (producing secretion of ACTH) or a malignancy elsewhere, e.g. in the lung, or adrenal gland requiring extensive therapy with corticosteroid drugs. Symptoms include obesity, reddening of face and neck, growth of body and facial hair, OSTEOPOROSIS, high blood pressure and possible mental disturbances.

cuticle a name for the outer layer or EPIDERMIS of the skin. Also refers to the outer layer of cells covering a hair.

cyanide poisoning poisoning with any salts of hydrocyanic acid which paralyses the nervous system and is usually fatal within minutes.

cyanocobalamin *see* VITAMIN B12.

cyanosis a blue appearance of the skin due to insufficient oxygen within the blood. It is first noticeable on the lips, tips of the ears, cheeks and nails and occurs in heart failure, lung diseases, asphyxia and in 'blue babies' who have congenital heart defects.

cystic fibrosis a genetic disease, the defective gene responsible for it being located on human chromosome no. 7. The disease affects all the mucus-secreting glands of the lungs, pancreas, mouth and gastrointestinal tract and also the sweat glands of the skin. A thick mucus is produced which affects the production of pancreatic enzymes and cause the bronchi to widen (bronchiectasis) and become clogged. Respiratory infections are common and the sweat contains abnormally high levels of sodium and chloride. The stools also contain a lot of mucus and have a foul smell. The disease is incurable and cannot be diagnosed by antenatal tests.

cystitis inflammation of the bladder

normally caused by bacterial infection, the causal organism usually being *E. coli*. It is marked by the need to pass urine frequently accompanied by a burning sensation. There may be cramp-like pains in the lower abdomen with dark strong urine which contains blood. The condition is common in females and is usually not serious, but there is a danger that the infection may spread to the kidneys.

cysts small, usually benign, tumours containing fluid (or soft secretions) within a membranous sac. Examples are wens (caused by blockage of sebaceous glands in the skin), cysts in the breasts caused by blocked milk ducts and ovarian cysts which may be large and contain a clear, thick liquid. *Dermoid cysts* are congenital and oc-cur at sites in the body where embryonic clefts have closed up before birth. These may contain fatty substances, hair, skin fragments of bone and even teeth. *Hydatid cysts* are a stage in the life cycle of certain parasites (tapeworm) and may be found in man, especially in the liver.

cytoplasm the substance within the cell wall that surrounds the nucleus and contains a number of organelles.

cytotoxic a substance which damages or destroys cells. Cytotoxic drugs are used in the treatment of various forms of cancer and act by inhibiting cell division. They also damage normal cells and their use has to be carefully regulated in each individual patient. They may be used in combination with RADIOTHERAPY or on their own.

D

dead space the volume of air, primarily in the TRACHEA and bronchi, that does not take part in the oxygen/carbon dioxide exchange. In each breath taken into the lungs, this proportion does not contribute directly to the respiratory process.

deafness a partial or complete loss of hearing. The deafness may be temporary or permanent, conductive or sensory, congenital or acquired. Congenital hearing loss is not a common cause. In many cases, the loss is due to a problem in the cochlea, the auditory nerve or the brain-nerve deafness. This is a common condition in the elderly although no particular cause can be identified. Other causes include exposure to industrial noise or explosions.

Conductive hearing loss is due to poor transmission of sound waves to the inner ear, possibly due to OTITIS which can cause middle ear inflammation and perforation of the ear drum. This latter condition can be treated by surgery or the use of a hearing aid.

decidua the soft epithelial tissue that forms a lining to the uterus during pregnancy and which is shed at birth.

defibrillation the application of a large electric shock to the chest wall of a patient whose heart is fibrillating (*see* FIBRILLATION). The delivery of a direct electric countershock hopefully allows the pacemaker to set up the correct rhythm again.

degeneration the deterioration over time of body tissues or an organ resulting in a lessening of its function. The changes may be structural or chemical and there are a number of types: fatty, FIBROID, calcareous (as with CONCRETIONS), mucoid and so on. Degeneration may be due to ageing, heredity or poor nutrition. Poisons such as alcohol also contribute to degeneration, as with CIRRHOSIS.

dehydration the removal of water. More specifically, the loss of water from the body through diuresis, sweating etc. or a reduction in water content due to a low intake. Essential body electrolytes (such as sodium chloride and potassium) are disrupted and after the first symptom, thirst, irritability and confusion follow.

delirium a mental disorder typified by confusion, agitation, fear, anxiety, illusions and sometimes hallucinations. The causal cerebral disfunction may be due to deficient nutrition, stress, toxic poisoning or mental shock.

delirium tremens a form of DELIRIUM due often to partial or total withdrawal of alcohol after a period of excessive intake. Symptoms are varied and include insomnia, agitation, confusion and fever, often with vivid hallucinations.

delta waves one of the four types of brain waves and the slowest of the four. Delta waves are associated with deep sleep. If delta waves are seen in the *electroencephalogram* of a waking adult, brain damage is indicated e.g. as with epileptics and around brain tumours.

deltoid the muscle, triangular in shape, that covers the shoulder and is attached to the collar bone, shoulder blade and humerus. It enables the arm to be raised from the side.

dementia a mental disorder typified by confusion, disorientation, memory loss, personality changes and a lessening of intellectual capacity. Dementia occurs in several forms: SENILE DEMENTIA, ALZHEIMER'S DISEASE and MULTI-INFARCT DEMENTIA. The causes are various and include vascular disease, brain tumour, SUBDURAL HAEMATOMA, HYDROCEPHALUS and hyperthyroidism.

demyelination the process whereby the myelin sheath surrounding a nerve fibre is destroyed, resulting in impaired nerve function. This is associated with MULTIPLE SCLEROSIS but can also happen after a nerve has been injured.

denaturation the disruption, usually by heat, of the weak bonds that hold a protein together. Extremes of temperature are fatal to most animals because the ENZYMES (which are proteins) that perform essential catalytic functions in life-sustaining biochemical processes, are irreversibly denatured.

dendrite one of numerous thin branching extensions of a nerve cell. The dendrites are at the 'receiving end' of the nerve cell (neuron) and they form a network which increases the area for receiving impulses from the terminals of axons of other neurons at the SYNAPSE.

dentine the material which forms the bulk of a tooth, lying between the pulp cavity and the enamel. It is similar to bone in composition but contains blood capillaries, nerve fibres and extensions of odontoblasts (cells producing the dentine).

depressant a drug which is used to reduce the functioning of a system of the body e.g. a respiratory depressant. Drugs such as opiates, general anaesthetics, etc. are depressants.

depression a mental state of extreme sadness dominated by pessimism and in which normal behaviour patterns (sleep, appetite, etc.) are disturbed. Causes are varied: upsetting events, loss, etc. and treatment involves the use of therapy and drugs.

dermatitis an inflammation of the skin which is similar in many respects to, and often interchanged with, ECZEMA. It is characterized by erythema (redness due to dilatation of capillaries near the surface), pain and PRURITIS. Several forms of dermatitis can be identified: Contact dermatitis caused by the skin coming into contact with a substance to which the skin is sensitive. A large range of compounds and materials may cause such a reaction. Treatment usually involves the use of a corticosteroid. Light dermatitis manifests itself as a reddening and blistering of skin exposed to sunlight and this occurs on hands, face and neck and occurs during the summer months. Some individuals become sensitized by drugs or perfumes in cosmetics while others have an in-

nate sensitivity. Erythroderma or exfoliative dermatitis involves patches of reddened skin which thicken and peel off. It is often associated with other skin conditions, e.g. PSORIASIS. Corticosteroids form a central part of the treatment in this case.

desensitization the technique whereby an individual builds up resistance to an allergen by taking gradually increasing doses of the allergen over a period of time. Also in the treatment of phobias, where a patient is gradually faced with the thing that is feared and concurrently learns to relax and reduce anxiety.

detached retina when the retina becomes detached from the choroid (a layer of the eyeball with blood vessels and pigment that absorbs excess light, preventing blurred vision). The detachment may be due to tumour or inflammation, or to the leaking of vitreous humour through holes in the retina to fill the space between retina and choroid thus disrupting the fine attachments. The condition can be corrected by surgery whereby heat binds the retina and choroid together using scarred tissue.

diabetes insipidus a rare condition which is completely different from DIABETES MELLITUS and is characterized by excessive thirst (*see* POLYDIPSIA) and POLYURIA. It is due to a lack of the antidiuretic hormone or the inability of the kidney to respond to the hormone.

diabetes mellitus a complex metabolic disorder involving carbohydrate, fat and protein. It results in an accumulation of sugar in the blood and urine and is due to a lack of INSULIN produced by the pancreas, so that sugars are not broken down to release energy. Fats are thus used as an alternative energy source. Symptoms include thirst, POLYURIA, loss of weight and the use of fats can produce KETOSIS and KETONURIA. In its severest form, convulsions are followed by a diabetic coma.

Treatment relies upon dietary control with doses of insulin or drugs, long-term effects include thickening of the arteries, and in some cases the eyes, kidneys, nervous system, skin and circulation may be affected (*see also* HYPOGLYCAEMIA and HYPERGLYCAEMIA).

diagnosis the process whereby a particular disease or condition is identified after consideration of the relevant parameters, viz.: symptoms, physical manifestations, results from laboratory tests and so on. In many instances the diagnosis requires greater skills than does the treatment.

dialysis the use of a semipermeable membrane to separate large and small molecules by selective diffusion. Starch and proteins are large molecules while salts, glucose and amino acids are small molecules. If a mixture of large and small molecules is separated from distilled water by a semipermeable membrane, the smaller molecules diffuse into the water which is itself replenished. This principle is the basis of the artificial kidney which, because a patient's blood is processed, is known as HAEMODIALYSIS.

diaphragm a membrane of muscle and tendon that separates the thoracic and abdominal cavities. It is covered by a SEROUS MEMBRANE and attached at the lower ribs, breast-bone and backbone. The diaphragm is important in breathing, when it bulges up to its resting position during exhalation. It flattens during inhalation and in so doing it reduces pressure in the thoracic cavity and helps to draw air into the lungs.

Also a rubber bowl-shaped cap used as a contraceptive with spermicidal cream. It fits inside the VAGINA over the neck of the UTERUS.

diaphysis the central part of shaft of a long bone.

diarrhoea increased frequency and looseness of bowel movement, involving the passage of unusually soft faeces. Diarrhoea can be caused by food poisoning, COLITIS, IRRITABLE BOWEL SYNDROME, DYSENTERY, etc. A severe case will result in the loss of water and salts which must be replaced and anti-diarrhoeal drugs are used in certain circumstances.

diastase (amylases) ENZYMES that break down starch into sugar. Specifically, diastase is the part of malt containing â amylase. Diastase is used to help in the digestion of starch in some digestive disorders.

diastasis the separation of a growing bone from the shaft.

diastole the point at which the heart relaxes between contractions, when the ventricles fill with blood. This usually lasts about half a second at the end of which the ventricles are about three-quarters full.

diathermy the use of high-frequency non-lethal electric currents to produce heat in a part of the body. The heat generated increases blood flow and is used for the relief of deep-seated pain such as NEURITIS, SCIATICA and particularly painful rheumatic conditions. The use of currents in this way can be adopted to cauterize tissues and small blood vessels (the latter because the blood coagulates on contact with the heated element).

dietetics the study and application of the science of nutrition to all aspects of food and feeding for individuals and groups in health and disease.

digestion the process of breaking down food into substances that can be absorbed and used by the body. Digestion begins with the chewing and grinding of food at which point it is mixed with saliva to commence the process of breakdown. Most digestion occurs in the stomach and small intestine. In the stomach the food is subject to gastric juice which contains pepsins to break down proteins and hydrochloric acid. The food is mixed and becomes totally soluble before passing into the small intestine as CHYME, where it is acted upon by pancreatic juice, bile, bacteria and succus entericus (intestinal juices).

Water is absorbed in the intestine in a very short time, while the bulk of the food may take several hours. The chyme forms chyle due to the action of bile and pancreatic juice. Fats are removed from this in emulsion form into the lymph vessels (*see* LACTEAL) and then into the blood. Sugars, salts and amino acids move directly into the small blood vessels in the intestine and the whole process is promoted by microfolding of the intestine wall producing finger-like projections (villi). The food passes down the intestine due to muscle contractions of the intestine wall and ultimately the residue and waste are excreted.

digitalis a powder derived from the leaf of the wild foxglove (*Digitalis purpurea*) and which finds use in cases of heart disease. It acts in two ways; strengthening each heart beat and increasing each pause (DIASTOLE) so that the damaged heart muscle has longer to rest. It also has a diuretic effect. Digitalis poisoning may occur with prolonged use or an overdose. Symptoms include vomiting, nausea, blurred vision, irregular heartbeat and possible breathing difficulties and unconsciousness.

dilatation and curettage (D & C) the technique whereby the cervix is opened using DILATORS and then the lining is scraped using a curette. Such sampling is performed for the removal of incomplete abortions and tumours, to diagnose disease of the uterus or to correct bleeding, etc.

dilator an instrument employed to increase the opening of an orifice. Also, a muscle that increases the diameter of a vessel, or organ. The same term is applied to drugs that achieve a similar effect.

diphtheria an infectious disease caused by the bacterium *Corynebacterium diphtheriae,* and commonest in children. The infection causes a membranous lining on the throat which can interfere with breathing and eating. The toxin produced by the bacterium damages heart tissue and the central nervous system and it can be fatal if not treated. The infection is countered by injection of the antitoxin with penicillin or erythromycin taken to kill the bacterium. Diphtheria can be immunized against.

diplegia paralysis on both sides of the body.

diplopia double vision. It is caused by disfunction in the muscles that move the eyeballs such that rays of light fall in different places on the two retinae. The condition can be due to a nervous disease, intoxication or certain diseases such as diphtheria.

disc a flattened circular structure, such as the cartilage between vertebrae.

disinfection the process of killing PATHOGENIC organisms (not spores) to prevent the spread of infection. Different compounds are used, appropriate to the surface being disinfected.

dislocation injuries to joints such that bones are displaced from their normal, respective positions. Associated effects include bruising of the surrounding tissues and tearing of the ligaments that hold the bones together. Most dislocations are simple rather than compound (the latter being where the bone punctures the skin), and acquired rather than CONGENITAL. Immediate treatment involves the application of a splint or bandage to render the joint stable. Repositioning the bone (REDUCTION) requires skill, after which the limb must be fixed to avoid a repetition. Even after some time, care is necessary when using the limb.

diuresis an increase in urine production due to disease, drugs, hormone imbalance or increased fluid intake.

diuretica a substance that increases urine formation and excretion and which may work specifically within the kidney e.g. by prevention of sodium, and therefore water, reabsorption or outside the kidney.

diverticulitis the inflammation of diverticula (*see* DIVERTICULUM) in the large intestine. During the condition, there are cramp-like pains in the left side of the abdomen, possibly with constipation and fever. Treatment normally involves complete rest with no solid food, and antibiotics.

diverticulosis the condition in which there are DIVERTICULA in the large intestine, occurring primarily in the lower colon. They are caused by the muscles of the bowel forcing the bowel out through weak points in the wall. It is thought that it may be related to diet, but symptoms are not always produced.

diverticulum in general, a pouch extending from a main cavity. Specifically applied to the intestine, a sac-like protrusion through the wall, many of which usually develop later in life. The formation of diverticula is DIVERTICULOSIS and their inflammation, DIVERTICULITIS.

DNA (deoxyribonucleic acid) a nucleic acid and the primary constituent of CHROMOSOMES. It transmits genetic information from parents to offspring in the form of GENES. It is a very large molecule comprising two twisted nucleotide chains which can store enormous amounts of information in a stable but not rigid way i.e. parental traits and characteristics are passed on but evolutionary changes are allowed to occur.

donor insemination *see* ARTIFICIAL INSEMINATION.

donor a person who donates part of his/her body for use in other people. Blood is the most common donation but many tissues and organs are now used including kidneys, livers, hearts, skin corneas, bone marrow etc. Organ donations occur when the donor has been certified as brainstem dead (*see* BRAINSTEM DEAD).

dopa an amino acid compound formed from tyrosine (an amino acid synthesized in the body) and which is a precursor of DOPAMINE and NORADRENALINE (norepinephrine in America). A drug form, levodopa or l-dopa, is used to treat PARKINSONISM, as it can increase the concentration of dopamine in the basal ganglia.

dopamine a catecholamine derived from DOPA and an intermediate in the synthesis of NORADRENALINE. (Catecholamines comprise benzene, hydroxyl groups and an amine group and are physiologically important in the functioning of the nervous system, mainly as NEUROTRANSMITTERS). It is found mainly in the basal ganglia of the brain and a deficiency is typical in PARKINSONISM.

dosage the overall amount of a drug administered, determined by size, frequency and number of doses and taking into account the patient's age, weight and possible allergic reactions. Modern techniques enable controlled dosage using transdermals (drugs absorbed from a plaster on the skin) and implantable devices. The latter are polymeric substances containing the drug and placed just beneath the skin which deliver the correct dose at any predetermined rate.

Down's syndrome (formerly called mongolism) a syndrome created by a CONGENITAL CHROMOSOME disorder which occurs as an extra chromosome 21, producing 47 in each body cell. Characteristic facial features are produced - a shorter, broader face with slanted eyes (similar to the Mongolian races, hence the term mongolism). It also results in a shorter stature, weak muscles and the possibility of heart defects and respiratory problems. The syndrome also confers mental retardation.

Down's syndrome occurs once in approximately 600 to 700 live births and although individuals may live beyond middle age, life expectancy is reduced and many die in infancy. The incidence increases with the age of the mother from 0.04% of children to women under 30 to 3% to women at 45. It is therefore likely that above 35 an AMNIOCENTESIS test would be made.

drug clearance is defined as the volume of blood which in one minute is completely cleared of a drug.

drug interactions when a patient is prescribed several drugs, there is the possibility for interactions between some or all of the medications. There are several ways in which the interaction may occur e.g. one drug displacing another at the site of action thus affecting its effectiveness; as alteration in the rate of destruction of one drug by another (by altering the activity of liver enzymes); prevention of absorption.

duct a narrow tube-like structure joining a gland with an organ or the body surface, through which a secretion passes e.g. sweat ducts opening onto the skin.

ductless gland a gland which releases the secretion directly into the blood for transport around the body, e.g. the pituitary and thyroid. Some glands, such as the PANCREAS, operate as a ductless gland (for INSULIN), but secrete a digestive juice via ducts into the small intestine.

ductus arteriosus when a foetus is in the uterus, the lungs do not function and the foetal blood bypasses the lungs by means of the ductus arteriosus which takes blood from the pulmonary artery to the aorta. The vessel stops functioning soon after birth.

duodenal ulcer the commonest type of PEPTIC ULCER. Duodenal ulcers may occur after the age of 20 and are more common in men. The cause is open to debate but probably results from an abrasion or break in the duodenum lining which is then exacerbated by gastric juice. Smoking seems to be a contributory but not causal factor.

The ulcer manifests itself as an upper abdominal pain roughly two hours after a meal that also occurs during the night. Food (e.g. milk) relieves the symptom and a regime of frequent meals and milky snacks, with little or no fried food and spices and a minimum of strong tea and coffee is usually adopted. Recent drug treatments enable the acid secretion to be reduced, thus allowing the ulcer to heal. Surgery is required only if there is no response to treatment, if the PYLORUS is obstructed or if the ulcer becomes perforated. The latter is treated as an emergency.

duodenum the first part of the small intestine where food (CHYME) from the stomach is subject to action by BILE and pancreatic enzymes. The duodenum also secretes a hormone secretion that contributes to the breakdown of fats, proteins and carbohydrates. In the duodenum, the acid conditions pertaining from the stomach are neutralized and rendered alkaline for the intestinal enzymes to operate.

dura mater *see* MENINGES and BRAIN.

dwarfism an abnormal underdevelopment of the body manifested by small stature. There are several causes including incorrect functioning of the PITUITARY or THYROID glands. Pituitary dwarfism produces a small but correctly proportioned body and if diagnosed sufficiently early, treatment with growth hormone can help. A defect in the thyroid gland may results in CRETINISM or in the activity of digestive organs and their secretions. RICKETS may also be responsible for dwarfism.

dysarthria poorly articulated speech which sounds weak or slurred due to impairment of the control of muscles that effect speech. The cause may be damage in the brain or to the muscles themselves. Dysarthria occurs with strokes, multiple sclerosis, cerebral palsy and so on.

dysentery an infection and ulceration of the lower part of the bowels that causes severe diarrhoea with the passage of mucus and blood. There are two forms of dysentery caused by different organisms. Amoebic dysentery is due to *Entamoeba histolytica* which is spread via infected food or water and occurs mainly in the tropics and sub-tropics. The appearance of symptoms may be delayed but in addition to diarrhoea there is indigestion, anaemia and weight loss. Drugs are used in treatment.

Bacillary dysentery is caused by the bacterium *Shigella* and spreads by contact with a carrier or contaminated food. Symptoms appear from one to six days after infection and include diarrhoea, cramp, nausea, fever and the severity of the attack varies. Antibiotics may be given to kill the bacteria but recovery usually occurs within one to two weeks.

dyslexia a disorder that renders reading or learning to read difficult. There is usually an associated problem in writing and spelling correctly. A very small number of children are affected severely and boys are more prone than girls by a factor of three.

dyspepsia (or indigestion) after eating there may be discomfort in the upper abdomen/lower chest with heartburn, nausea and flatulence accompanying a feeling of fullness.

The causes are numerous and include GALLSTONES, PEPTIC ULCER, HIATUS HERNIA and diseases of the liver or pancreas.

dysphasia a general term for an impairment of speech whether it is manifested as a difficulty in understanding language or in self-expression. There is a range of conditions with varying degrees of severity. *Global aphasia* is a total inability to communicate, however some individuals partially understand what is said to them. *Dysphasia* is when thoughts can be expressed up to a point. *Non-fluent dysphasia* represents poor self-expression but good understanding while the reverse is called *fluent dysphasia*. The condition may be due to a stroke or other brain damage and can be temporary or permanent.

E

ear the sense organ used for detection of sound and maintenance of balance. It comprises three parts, the external or outer, middle and inner ear, the first two acting to collect sound waves and transmit them to the inner ear, where the hearing and balance mechanisms are situated.

The outer ear (*auricle* or *pinna*) is a cartilage and skin structure which is not actually essential to hearing in man. The middle ear is an air-filled cavity that is linked to the PHARYNX

via the EUSTACHIAN TUBE. Within the middle ear are the ear (or auditory) ossicles, three bones called the *incus, malleus* and *stapes* (anvil, hammer and stirrup respectively). Two small muscles control the bones and the associated nerve (the chorda tympani). The ossicles bridge the middle ear, connecting the eardrum with the inner ear and in so doing convert sound (air waves) into mechanical movements which then impinge upon the fluid of the inner ear.

The inner ear lies within the temporal bone of the skull and contains the apparatus for hearing and balance. The COCHLEA is responsible for hearing and balance is maintained by the semicircular canals. The latter are made up of three loops positioned mutually at right angles and in each is the fluid endolymph. When the head is moved the fluid moves accordingly and sensory cells produce impulses that are transmitted to the brain.

earache pain in the ear may be due directly to inflammation of the middle ear but is often referred pain from other conditions, e.g. infections of the nose, larynx or tooth decay.

eating disorders *see* ANOREXIA and BULIMIA.

ECG *see* ELECTROCARDIOGRAM.

echocardiography the use of ULTRASOUND to study the heart and its movements.

echography (or ultrasonography) the use of sound waves (ULTRASOUND) to create an image of the deeper structures of the body, based upon the differences in reflection of the sound by various parts of the body.

eclampsia convulsions that occur during pregnancy, usually at the later stages or during delivery. Although the cause is not known the start of convulsions may be associated with cerebral OEDEMA or a sudden rise in blood pressure. Kidney function is usually badly affected. The condition is often preceded for days or weeks by symptoms such as headache, dizziness and vomiting and seizures follow. The fits differ in severity and duration and in the one in twelve fatalities, there may be a cerebral haemorrhage, pneumonia or the breathing may gradually fade. The condition requires immediate treatment as it threatens both mother and baby. Treatment is by drugs and reduction of outside stimuli, and a CAESARIAN section is undertaken.

ectopic referring to something or some event that is not in its usual place or occurring at its usual time e.g. an ectopic pregnancy is one that is outside the uterus.

eczema an inflammation of the skin that causes itching, a red rash and often small blisters that weep and become encrusted. This may be followed by the skin thickening and then peeling off in scales. There are several types of eczema, *atopic* being one of the most common. (Atopic is the hereditary tendency to form allergic reactions due to an antibody in the skin). A form of atopic eczema is infantile eczema that starts in 3 or 4 months and it is often the case that eczema, hay fever and asthma is found in the family history. However, many children improve markedly as they approach the age of 10 or 11. The treatment for such conditions usually involves the use of HYDROCORTISONE and other steroid creams and ointments.

EEG *see* ELECTROENCEPHALOGRAM.

ejaculation the emission of semen from the penis via the urethra. It is a reflex action produced during copulation or masturbation and the sensation associated with it is orgasm.

electrocardiogram a record of the changes in the heart's electrical potential, on an instrument called an electrocardiograph. The subject is connected to the equipment by leads on the chest and legs or arms. A normal trace has one wave for the activity of the atria and others relating to the ventricular beat. Abnormal heart activity is often indicated in the trace and it therefore forms a useful diagnostic aid.

electroencephalogram (EEG) a record of the brain's electrical activity measured on an electroencephalograph. Electrodes on the scalp record the charge of electric potential - or brain waves. There are four main types of waves: alpha, beta, theta and delta. Alpha waves, with a frequency of ten per second, occur when awake and delta waves (seven or less per second) occur in sleeping adults. The occurrence of delta waves in wakeful adults indicates brain damage or cerebral tumours.

elephantiasis a dramatic and debilitating enlargement of skin and underlying connective tissue due to inflammation of the skin, subcutaneous tissue and the blocking of lymph vessels, preventing drainage. Inflammation and blocking of vessels is due to parasitic worms - filariae which are carried to man by mosquitoes. The parts of the body most commonly affected are the legs, scrotum and breasts, in some cases to enormous proportions. The associated muscles of a limb may degenerate due to the abnormal pressure on them, and eventually overall health suffers. Prevention is the key, by eradication of the mosquitoes, but some relief is gained by using certain drugs early in the history of the disease.

embolectomy the surgical, and often emergency, removal of an EMBOLUS

or clot to clear an arterial obstruction.

embolism the state in which a small blood vessel is blocked by an EMBOLUS, or fragment of material which the circulatory system has carried through larger vessels. This plug may be fragments of a clot, a mass of bacteria, air bubbles that have entered the system during an operation, or a fragment of tumour. The blockage leads usually to the destruction of that part of the organ supplied by the vessel. The most common case is a pulmonary embolism.

embolus material carried by the blood which then lodges elsewhere in the body (*see* EMBOLISM). The material may be a blood clot, fat, air, a piece of tumour etc.

embryo the stage of development from 2 weeks, when the fertilized ovum is implanted in the uterus, to 2 months.

embryology the study of the embryo, its growth and development from fertilization to birth.

embryo transfer (*see also* IN VITRO FERTILIZATION) the fertilization of an ovum by sperm and its development into an early embryo, outside the mother, and its subsequent implantation in the mother's uterus. Such procedures result in what is popularly termed a 'test-tube baby.'

emesis is the medical term for vomit.

emetics a substance that causes vomiting. Direct emetics such as mustard in water, copper sulphate, alum or a lot of salty water irritate the stomach, while indirect emetics such as apomorphine and ipecacuanha act on the centre of the brain that controls the act of vomiting. Tickling the throat is also classed as an emetic (indirect). Emetics tend to be used little nowadays, but great care must be exercised if their use is advocated.

emollients substances that soften or soothe the skin whether in the form of a powder, oil or preparation, often used in the treatment of eczema. Examples are olive oil, and glycerin.

emphysema refers, in the main, to an abnormal condition of the lungs where the walls of the are over-inflated and distended and changes in their structure occur. This destruction of parts of the walls produces large air-filled spaces which do not contribute to the respiratory process. Acute cases of emphysema may be caused by whooping cough, bronchopneumonia and chronic cases often accompany chronic bronchitis which itself is due in great part to smoking. Emphysema is also developed after tuberculosis when the lungs are stretched until the fibres of the alveolar walls are destroyed. Similarly in old age, the alveolar membrane may collapse producing large air sacs, with decreased surface area.

encephalins peptides that act as NEUROTRANSMITTERS. Two have been identified, both acting as analgesics when their release controls pain. They are found in the brain and in nerve cells of the spinal cord.

encephalitis inflammation of the brain. It is usually a viral infection and sometimes occurs as a complication of some common infectious diseases, e.g. measles or chickenpox. There are several forms of the disease including *Encephalitis lethargica* (sleepy sickness or epidemic encephalitis) which attacks and causes swelling in the basal ganglia, cerebrum and brain stem that may result in tissue destruction; Japanese encephalitis, which is caused by a virus carried by mosquitoes and tick-borne encephalitis which occurs in Europe and Siberia. In most cases there is no readily available treatment under the causative virus is *Herpes*.

encephalography any technique used to record brain structure or activity e.g. electroencephalography (*see* ELECTROENCEPHALOGRAM).

encephaloid the term given to a form of cancer that superficially resembles brain tissue.

encephalomyelitis inflammation of the brain and spinal cord typified by headaches, fever, stiff neck and back pain, with vomiting. Depending upon the extent of the inflammation and the patient's condition, encephalomyelitis may cause paralysis, personality changes, coma or death.

encephalopathy any disease affecting the brain or an abnormal condition of the brain's structure and function. It refers in particular to degenerative and chronic conditions such as Wernicke's encephalopathy which is caused by a THIAMINE deficiency and associated with alcoholism.

endemic the term used to describe, for example, a disease that is indigenous to a certain area.

endocarditis inflammation of the ENDOCARDIUM, heart valves and muscle, caused by a bacterium, virus or rheumatic fever. Those at greatest risk are patients with some damage to the endocardium from a CONGENITAL deformity or alteration of the immune system by drugs. Patients suffer fever, heart failure and/or EMBOLISM.

Large doses of an antibiotic are used in treatment and surgery may prove necessary to repair heart valves that become damaged. If not treated the condition is fatal.

endocardium a fine membrane lining the heart and which forms a continuous membrane with the lining of veins and arteries. At the cavities of the heart it forms cusps at the valves and its surface is very smooth to facilitate blood flow.

endocrine glands DUCTLESS GLANDS that produce HORMONES for secretion directly into the bloodstream (or lymph). Some organs e.g. the PANCREAS also release secretions via a DUCT. In addition to the pancreas the major endocrine glands are the THYROID, PITUITARY, PARATHYROID, OVARY and TESTIS. Imbalances in the secretions of endocrine glands produce a variety of diseases (*see individual entries*).

endogenous referring to within the body, whether growing within, or originating from within or due to internal causes.

endometriosis the occurrence of ENDOMETRIUM in other parts of the body e.g. within the muscle of the uterus, in the ovary, FALLOPIAN TUBES, PERITONEUM and possibly the bowel. Because of the nature of tissue, it acts in a way similar to that of the uterus lining and causes pelvic pain, bleeding, painful menstruation. The condition occurs between puberty and the menopause and ceases during pregnancy. The treatment required may include total hysterectomy, but occasionally the administration of a steroid hormone will alleviate the symptoms.

endometritis inflammation of the ENDOMETRIUM caused commonly by bacteria but can also be due to a virus, parasite or foreign body. It is associated with fever and abdominal pain and occurs most after abortion or childbirth or women with an INTRAUTERINE CONTRACEPTIVE DEVICE.

endometrium the womb's mucous membrane lining that changes in structure during the menstrual cycle, becoming thicker with an increased blood supply later in the cycle. This is in readiness for receiving an embryo but if this does not happen, the endometrium breaks down and most is lost in menstruation.

endorphins a group of compounds, PEPTIDES that occur in the brain and have pain-relieving qualities similar to morphine. They are derived from a substance in the PITUITARY and are involved in endocrine control. In addition to their opiate effects, they are involved in urine output, depression of respiration, sexual activity and learning (*see also* ENCEPHALINS).

endoscope the general term for an instrument used to inspect the interior of a body cavity or organ, e.g. the gastroscope is for viewing the stomach. The instrument is fitted with lenses and a light source and is usually inserted through a natural opening although an incision can be used.

enema the procedure of putting fluid into the rectum for purposes of cleansing or therapy. An evacuant enema removes faeces and consists of soap in water or olive oil while a barium enema is given to permit an X-ray of the colon to be taken. The compound barium sulphate is opaque to X-rays. The insertion of drugs into the rectum is a therapeutic enema.

engagement the stage in a pregnancy

when the presenting part of the foetus which is usually the head, descends into the pelvis of the mother.

enteral the term meaning relating to the intestine.

enteral feeding the procedure of feeding a patient who is very ill through a tube via the nose, to the stomach. Through the tube is given a liquid, low waste food and there are a number of proprietary brands, some containing whole protein, some amino acids.

enteric fevers *see* TYPHOID FEVER and PARATYPHOID FEVER.

enteritis inflammation of the intestine, due usually to a viral or bacterial infection, causing diarrhoea.

enterovirus a virus that enters the body via the gut where it multiplies and from where they attack the central nervous system. Examples are POLIOMYELITIS and the Coxsackie viruses (the cause of severe throat infections, MENINGITIS, and inflammation of heart tissue, some muscles and the brain).

enzyme any protein molecule that acts as a catalyst in the biochemical processes of the body. They are essential to life ad are highly specific, acting on certain substrates at a set temperature and pH. Examples are the digestive enzymes amylase, lipase and trypsin. Enzymes act by providing active sites (one or more for each enzyme) to which substrate molecules bind, forming a short-lived intermediate. The rate of reaction is increased, and after the product is formed, the active site is freed. Enzymes are easily rendered inactive by heat and some chemicals. The names of most enzymes end in -*ase*, and this is added onto the name

of the substrate thus a peptidase breaks down peptides. Enzymes are vital for the normal functioning of the body and their lack or inactivity can produce metabolic disorders.

epidemic a disease that affects a large proportion of the population at the same time. Usually an infectious disease that occurs suddenly and spreads rapidly, e.g. today there are influenza epidemics.

epidermis the outer layer of the skin which comprises four layers and overlies the dermis. The top three layers are continually renewed as cells from the innermost germinative layer (called *the Malpighian layer or stratum germinativum*) are pushed outwards. The topmost layer (*stratum corneum*) is made up of dead cells where the CYTOPLASM has been replaced by KERATIN. This layer is thickest on the palms and soles of the feet.

epidural anaesthesia anaesthesia in the region of the pelvis, abdomen or genitals produced by local anaesthetic injected into the epidural space of the spinal column (the epidural space is that space between the vertebral canal and the dura mater of the spinal cord).

epiglottis situated at the base of the tongue, a thin piece of cartilage enclosed in MUCOUS MEMBRANE that covers the LARYNX. It prevents food from passing into the larynx and TRACHEA when swallowing. The epiglottis resembles a leaf in shape.

epiglottitis inflammation of the mucous membrane of the EPIGLOTTIS. Swelling of the tissues may obstruct the airway and swift action may be necessary i.e. a TRACHEOSTOMY to avoid a fatality. The other symptoms of epiglottitis are sore throat, fever, a croup-like cough and it occurs mainly in children, usually during the winter.

epilepsy a neurological disorder involving convulsions, seizures and loss of consciousness. There are many possible causes or associations of epilepsy, including cerebral trauma, brain tumour, cerebral haemorrhage and metabolic imbalances as in HYPOGLYCAEMIA. Usually an epileptic attack occurs without warning, with complete unconsciousness and some muscle contraction and spasms. Some drugs are used in treatment although little can be done during the fit itself.

epiphysis the softer end of a long bone that is separated from the shaft by a plate (the epiphyseal plate) of cartilage. It develops separately from the shaft but when the bone stops growing it disappears as the head and shaft fuse. Separation of the epiphysis is a serious fracture because the growing bone may be affected.

episiotomy the process of making an incision in the PERINEUM to enlarge a woman's vaginal opening to facilitate delivery of a child. The technique is used to prevent tearing of the perineum.

epithelioma an epithelial (*see* EPITHELIUM) tumour used formerly to describe any carcinoma.

epithelium (*plural* **epithelia**) tissue made up of cells packed closely together and bound by connective material. It covers the outer surface of the body and lines vessels and organs in the body. One surface is fixed to a basement membrane and the other is free and it provides a barrier against injury, microorganisms

and some fluid loss. There are various types of epithelium in single and multiple (or stratified) layers and differing shapes *viz.* cuboidal, squamous (like flat pads) and columnar. The shape suits the function thus the skin is formed from stratified squamous (and KERATINIZED) epithelium while columnar epithelia which can secrete solutions and absorb nutrients, line the intestines and stomach.

Epstein Barr virus the virus, similar to the herpes virus, that causes infectious mononucleosis (GLANDULAR FEVER) and is implicated in HEPATITIS.

erection the condition whereby erectile tissue in the penis (and to some degree the clitoris) is engorged with blood making it swell and become hard. It is due primarily to sexual arousal although it does occur during sleep, due to physical stimulation and it also occurs in young boys. It is a prerequisite of vaginal penetration for emission of semen.

erysipelas an infectious disease, caused by *Streptococcus pyogenes*. It produces an inflammation of the skin with associated redness. Large areas of the body may be affected and other symptoms may include vesicles, fever and pain with a feeling of heat and a tingling sensation. In addition to being isolated, patients are given penicillin.

erythema an inflammation or redness of the skin in which the tissues are congested with blood. The condition may be accompanied by pain or itching. There are numerous causes, some bacterial/viral and others physical e.g. mild sunburn.

erythroblast cells occurring in the red bone marrow that develop into red blood cells (called ERYTHRO-CYTES). The cells begin colourless but accumulate HAEMOGLOBIN and in mammals the nucleus is lost.

erythrocyte the red blood cell that is made in the bone marrow and occurs as a red disc, concave on both sides, full of HAEMOGLOBIN. These cells are responsible for carrying oxygen to tissues and carbon dioxide away

erythromycin an antibiotic used for bacterial and mycoplasmic infections. It is similar to penicillin in its activity and can be taken for infections that penicillin cannot be used to treat.

essential amino acid of the twenty amino acids required by the body, a number are termed essential because they must be in the diet as they cannot be synthesized in the body. The essential ones are: isoleucine, leucine, lysine, methionine, phenylalanine, threonine, tryptophan and valine. In addition, infants require arginine and histidine. A lack leads to protein deficiency, but they are available in meat, cheese and eggs, and all eight would be obtained if the diet contained corn and beans.

essential fatty acid there are three polyunsaturated acids in this category which cannot be produced in the body - arachidonic, linoleic and linolenic. These compounds are found in vegetable and fish oils and are vital in metabolism and proper functioning. A deficiency may cause such symptoms as allergic conditions, skin disorders, poor hair and nails and so on.

essential hypertension *see* HYPERTENSION.

etiology *see* AETIOLOGY.

eugenics the study of how the inherited characteristics of the human population can be improved by genetics or selective/controlled breeding.

euploid term meaning with a chromosome number that is an exact multiple of the normal (haploid) number.

eustachian tube tubes, one on each side, that connect the middle ear to the PHARYNX. The short (about 35 - 40mm) tube is fine at the centre and wider at both ends and is lined with mucous membrane. It is normally closed but opens to equalize air pressure on either side of the eardrum. It was named after the 16th century Italian anatomist Eustachio.

euthanasia intentionally hastening the death of someone who is suffering from a disease that is painful, incurable and inevitably fatal. The patient and/or their relatives consent to this whether it is achieved by administering a lethal drug or by withholding treatment.

Ewing's sarcoma a malignant bone cancer that develops from the marrow in the pelvis or long bones. It occurs in young adults and children and soon spreads around the body. It is uncommon but very malignant although recent use of anticancer drugs has prolonged the life expectancy of sufferers. The cancer was named after the American pathologist James Ewing.

excision in general terms, cutting out. More specifically the removal of, for example, a gland or tumour from the body.

excoriation injury of the surface of the skin (or other part of the body) caused by the abrasion or scratching of the area.

excreta waste material discharged

from the body. The term is often used specifically to denote faeces.

excretion the removal of all waste material from the body, including urine and faeces, the loss of water and salts through sweat glands, and the elimination of carbon dioxide and water vapour from the lungs.

exogenous originating outside the body, and can also refer to an organ of the body.

expectorants a group of drugs that are taken to help in the removal of secretions from the lungs, bronchi and trachea. The drugs work in one of several ways or can be used to combine their effects. Some dry up excess mucus and sputum while others render these secretions less viscous, to promote their removal. There are other varieties that work in still different ways.

extrasystole (*or* **ectopic beat**) a heart beat that is outside the normal rhythm of the heart and is due to an impulse generated outside the SINOATRIAL NODE. It may go unnoticed or it may seem that the heart has missed a beat. Extrasystoles are common in healthy people, but they may result from heart disease, or nicotine from smoking, or caffeine from excessive intake of tea and coffee. Drugs can be taken to suppress these irregular beats.

eye the complicated organ of sight. Each eye is roughly spherical and contained within the bony ORBIT in the skull. The outer layer is fibrous and comprises the opaque SCLERA and transparent CORNEA. The middle layer is vascular and is made up of the *choroid* (the blood supply for the outer half of the retina), *ciliary body* (which secretes aqueous humour) and the IRIS. The inner layer is sensory, the RETINA. Between the cornea and the LENS is a chamber filled with aqueous humour and behind the lens is a much larger cavity with vitreous humour. Light enters the eye through the cornea and thence via the aqueous humour to the lens which focuses the light onto the retina. The latter contains CONE and ROD cells which are sensitive to light and impulses are sent to the visual cortex of the brain via the optic nerve.

F

facial nerve the cranial nerve which has a number of branches and supplies the muscles which control facial expression. It also has branches to the middle ear, taste buds, salivary glands and lacrimal glands. Some branches are motor and others sensory in function.

facial paralysis paralysis of the facial nerve, which leads to a loss of function in the muscles of the face producing a lack of expression in the affected side. It occurs in the condition known as *Bell's palsy* in which there may also be a loss of taste and inability to close the eye. The condition is often temporary, if caused by inflammation which recovers in time. However, if the nerve itself is damaged by injury or if the person has suffered a stroke, the condition is likely to be permanent.

factor VIII this is one of the COAGULATION FACTORS normally present in the blood and is known as antihaemophilic factor. If the factor is deficient in males it results in HAEMOPHILIA.

faeces the end waste product of digestion which is formed in the colon and discharged from the bowels via the ANUS. Also known as stools, it consists of undigested food (chiefly cellulose), bacteria, mucus and other secretions, water and bile pigments which are responsible for the colour. The condition and colour of the faeces are indicators of general health e.g. pale stools are produced in JAUNDICE and COELIAC DISEASE and black stools often indicate the presence of digested blood.

fainting also known as *syncope*, this is a temporary and brief loss of consciousness caused by a sudden drop in the blood supply to the brain. It can occur in perfectly healthy people brought about by prolonged standing or emotional shock. It may also result from an infection, during pregnancy, from severe pain or loss of blood through injury. Fainting is often preceded by giddiness, blurred vision, sweating and ringing in the ears. Recovery is usually complete, producing no lasting ill-effects, although this depends upon the underlying cause.

Fallopian tubes a pair of tubes, one of which leads from each ovary to the womb. At the ovary, the tube is expanded to form a funnel with finger-like projections, known as fimbriae, surrounding the opening. This funnel does not communicate directly with the ovary but is open to the abdominal cavity. However, when an egg is released from the ovary the fimbriae move and waft it into the fallopian tube. The tube is about 10 to 12cm long and leads directly in to the womb at the lower end through a narrow opening.

false rib *see* RIB.

farmer's lung an allergic condition caused by sensitivity to inhaled dust and fungal spores that are found in mouldy hay or straw. It is a form of allergic alveolitis (inflammation of the ALVEOLI of the lungs) characterized by increasing breathlessness. The condition may be treated by CORTICOSTEROID drugs but can only be cured by avoidance of the allergen.

fascioliasis a disease of the liver and bile ducts caused by the organism *Fasciola hepatica* or liver fluke. Human beings and animals are hosts to the adult flukes and the eggs of the parasite are passed out in faeces. These are taken up by a certain species of snail which forms an intermediate host for the parasite, and from which the larval stages are deposited on vegetation, especially wild watercress. Human beings are then infected especially by eating wild watercress which should always be avoided.

Symptoms include fever, loss of

appetite, indigestion, nausea and vomiting, diarrhoea, abdominal pain, severe sweating and coughing. In severe cases the liver may be damaged and there may be jaundice and even death. Chemotherapy is required to kill the flukes, the principal drugs being chloroquine and bithionol.

fat *see* ADIPOSE TISSUE.

fatigue physical or mental tiredness following a prolonged period of hard work. Muscle fatigue resulting from hard exercise is caused by a build up of *lactic acid.* Lactic acid is produced in muscles (as an end product of the breakdown of GLYCOGEN to produce energy), and builds up when there is an insufficient supply of oxygen. The muscle is unable to work properly until a period of rest and restored oxygen supply enables the lactic acid to be removed.

fatty acids a group of organic compounds each consisting of a long, straight hydrocarbon chain and a terminal carboxylic acid (COOH) group. The length of the chain varies from one to nearly thirty carbon atoms and the chains may be *saturated* or *unsaturated.* Some fatty acids can be synthesized within the body but others, the ESSENTIAL FATTY ACIDS, must be obtained from food. Fatty acids have three major roles within the body.

(1) They are components of glycolipids (lipids containing carbohydrate) and phospholipids (lipids containing phosphate). These are of major importance in the structure of tissues and organs.

(2) Fatty acids are important constituents of triglycerides (lipids which have three fatty acid molecules joined to a glycerol molecule). They are stored in the cytoplasm of many cells and are broken down when required to yield energy. They are the form in which the body stores fat.

(3) Derivatives of fatty acids function as hormones and intracellular messengers.

favism an inherited disorder which takes the form of severe haemolytic ANAEMIA (destruction of red blood cells) brought on by eating broad beans. A person having this disorder is sensitive to a chemical present in the beans and also to certain drugs, particularly some antimalarial drugs. It is caused by the lack of a certain enzyme, glucose 6-phosphate dehydrogenase, which plays an important role in glucose metabolism. The defective gene responsible is passed on as a SEX-LINKED dominant characteristic and appears to persist in populations where it occurs, because it also confers increased resistance to malaria.

febrile having a FEVER.

Fehling's test a test, now replaced by more modern methods, for detecting the presence of sugar in the urine.

femoral describing the femur or area of the thigh e.g. femoral artery, vein, nerve and canal.

femur the thigh bone which is the long bone extending from the hip to the knee and is the strongest bone in the body. It is the weight-bearing bone of the body and fractures are common in old people who have lost bone mass. It articulates with the pelvic girdle at the upper end, forming the hip joint and at the lower end with the patella (knee cap) and tibia to form the knee joint.

fertilization the fusion of SPERM (-ATOZOON) and OVUM to form a *zygote* which then undergoes cell division to become an embryo. Fertilization in humans takes place high up in the FALLOPIAN TUBE near the ovary and the fertilized egg travels down and becomes implanted in the womb.

fever an elevation of body temperature above the normal which accompanies many diseases and infections. The cause of fever is the production by the body of endogenous pyrogen which acts on the thermo-regulatory centre in the hypothalamus of the brain. This responds by promoting mechanisms which increase heat generation and lessen heat loss, leading to a rise in temperature. Fever is the main factor in many infections caused by bacteria or viruses and results from toxins produced by the growth of these organisms. Examples of these *primary* or *specific* fevers are diphtheria, scarlet fever and typhoid fever. An *intermittent fever* describes a fluctuating body temperature, which commonly accompanies MALARIA, in which the temperature sometimes returns to normal. In a *remittent fever* there is also a fluctuating body temperature but this does not return to normal. In a *relapsing fever*, caused by bacteria of the genus *Borella*, transmitted by ticks or lice, there is a recurrent fever every 3 to 10 days following the first attack which lasts for about one week.

fibreoptic endoscopy a method of viewing internal structures such as the digestive tract and tracheo-bron-chial tree using fibreoptics. Fibreoptics uses illumination from a cold light source which is passed down a bundle of quartz fibres. The instruments used are highly flexible compared to the older form of endoscope and can be employed to illuminate structures which were formerly inaccessible. Using fibreoptic endoscopy, direct procedures can be carried out, such as BIOPSY and polypectomy (surgical removal of a POLYP).

fibrillation the rapid non-synchronized contraction or tremor of muscles in which individual bundles of fibres contract independently. It applies especially to heart muscle and disrupts the normal beating so that the affected part is unable to pump blood. Two types of fibrillation may occur depending upon which muscle is affected. Atrial fibrillation, often resulting from ATHEROSCLEROSIS or rheumatic heart disease, affects the muscles of the atria and is a common type of arrhythmia. The heart beat and pulse are very irregular and cardiac output is maintained by the contraction of the ventricles alone. With ventricular fibrillation the heart stops pumping blood so that this, in effect, is cardiac arrest. The patient requires immediate emergency resuscitation or death ensues within minutes.

fibrin the end product of the process of blood COAGULATION, comprising threads of insoluble protein formed from a soluble precursor, FIBRINOGEN, by the activity of the enzyme thrombin. Fibrin forms a network which is the basis of a blood clot, *see* COAGULATION.

fibrinogen a COAGULATION FACTOR

present in the blood which is a soluble protein and the precursor of FIBRIN, *see* COAGULATION.

fibrocystic disease of the pancreas *see* CYSTIC FIBROSIS.

fibroid a type of benign tumour found in the womb (uterus) composed of fibrous and muscular tissue and varying in size from one or two mm to a mass weighing several pounds. They more commonly occur in childless women and those over the age of thirty-five. Fibroids may present no problems but alternatively can be the cause of pain, heavy and irregular menstrual bleeding, urine retention or frequency of MICTURITION and sterility. Fibroids can be removed surgically but often the complete removal of the womb (HYSTERECTOMY) is carried out.

fibroma a benign tumour composed of fibrous tissue.

fibrosis the formation of thickened connective or scar tissue usually as a result of injury or inflammation. This may affect the lining of the ALVEOLI of the lungs (pulmonary interstitial fibrosis) and causes breathlessness. *See also* CYSTIC FIBROSIS.

fibrosarcoma a malignant tumour of connective tissue particularly found in the limbs and especially the legs.

fibrositis inflammation of fibrous connective tissue, muscles and muscle sheaths, particularly in the back, legs and arms causing pain and stiffness.

fibrous tissue a tissue type which occurs abundantly throughout the body. *White fibrous tissue* consists of collagen fibres, a protein with a high tensile strength and unyielding structure, that forms ligaments, sinews and scar tissue, and occurs in the skin. *Yellow fibrous tissue* is composed of the fibres of another protein, elastin. It is very elastic and occurs in ligaments which are subjected to frequent stretching, such as those in the back of the neck. It also occurs in arterial walls and in the walls of the alveoli (*see* ALVEOLUS), and in the dermis layer of the skin.

fibula the outer, thin, long bone which articulates with the larger tibia in the lower leg.

fissure a natural cleft or groove or abnormal break in the skin or mucous membrane e.g. an anal fissure.

fistula an abnormal opening between two hollow organs or between such an organ or gland and the exterior. These may arise during development so that a baby may be born with a fistula. Alternatively, they can be produced by injury, infection or as a complication following surgery. A common example is an anal fistula, which may develop if an abscess present in the rectum bursts and produces a communication through the surface of the skin. An operation is normally required to correct a fistula, but healing is further complicated in the case of an anal fistula because of the passage of waste material through the bowels.

fit any sudden convulsive attack; a general term which is applied to an epileptic seizure, convulsion or bout of coughing.

flap a section of tissue, usually skin, which is excised from the underlying tissues except for one thin strip (pedicle), which is left for blood and nervous supply. The flap is used to repair an injury at another site in the body, the free part being sutured into place. After about three weeks, when the healing process is well under way, the remaining strip is detached and sewn into place. Flaps are commonly used in plastic surgery and also following amputation of a limb. *See* SKIN GRAFTING.

flat foot an absence of the arch of the foot so that the inner edge lies flat on the ground. It may occur in children in whom the ligaments of the foot are soft, or in older, obese adults or those who stand for long periods. Treatment is by means of exercises, built-up footwear and, in extreme cases, surgery.

flatulence a build-up of gas in the stomach or bowels which is released through the mouth or anus.

flexion bending of a joint or the term may also be applied to an abnormal shape in a body organ.

flexor any muscle that causes a limb or other body part to bend.

flutter an abnormal disturbance of heart beat rhythm which may affect the atria or ventricles but is less severe than FIBRILLATION. The causes are the same as those of fibrillation and the treatment is also similar.

flux an excessive and abnormal flow from any of the natural openings of the body e.g. alvine flux which is diarrhoea.

foetus an unborn child after the eighth week of development.

follicle any small sac, cavity or secretory gland. Examples are hair follicles and the Graafian follicles of the ovaries in and from which eggs mature and are released.

fontanelle openings in the skull of newborn and young infants in whom

the bone is not wholly formed and the sutures are incompletely fused. The largest of these is the *anterior fontanelle* on the top of the head which is about 2.5cm square at birth.

The fontanelles gradually close as bone is formed and are completely covered by the age of 18 months. If a baby is unwell, for example with a fever, the fontanelle becomes tense. If an infant is suffering from diarrhoea and possibly dehydrated, the fontanelle is abnormally depressed.

food poisoning an illness of the digestive system caused by eating food contaminated by certain bacteria, viruses or by chemical poisons (insecticides) and metallic elements such as mercury or lead. Symptoms include vomiting, diarrhoea, nausea and abdominal pain and these may arise very quickly and usually within twenty-four hours. Bacteria are the usual cause of food poisoning and proliferate rapidly producing toxins which cause the symptoms of the illness. Those involved include members of the genera *Salmonella, Staphylococcus, Campylobacter* and also *Clostridium botulinum*, the causal organism of botulism. Food poisoning may be fatal, the old and the young being especially at risk.

foot the part of the lower limb below the ankle made up of eleven small bones and having a structure similar to that of the hand. The *talus*, which articulates with the leg bones and the *calcaneus*, which forms the heel, are the largest of these.

foramen a hole or opening which usually refers to those which occur in some bones. For example the *foramen magnum* is a large hole at the base of the skull (in the *occipital bone*) through which the spinal cord passes out from the brain.

forceps surgical instruments, of which there are many different types, which are used as pincers.

foreskin the *prepuce* which is a fold of skin growing over the end (glans) of the penis.

fossa a natural hollow or depression on the surface or within the body. Examples include the fossae within the skull which house different parts of the brain and the cubital fossa, a hollow at the front of the elbow joint.

fovea any small depression, often referring to the one which occurs in the RETINA of the EYE in which a large number of the light-sensitive cells called CONES are situated. It is the site of greatest visual acuity being the region in which the image is focused when the eyes are fixed on an object.

fracture any break in a bone which may be complete or incomplete. In a *simple fracture* (or *closed fracture*) the skin remains more or less intact but in a *compound fracture* (or *open fracture*) there is an open wound connecting the bone with the surface. This type of fracture is more serious as it provides a greater risk of infection and more blood loss. If a bone which is already diseased suffers a fracture, (such as often occurs in older women who have OSTEOPOROSIS), this is known as a *pathological fracture*. A *fatigue fracture* occurs in a bone which suffers recurrent, persistent stress, e.g. the *March fracture* sometimes seen in the second toe of soldiers after long marches. *See also* STRESS FRACTURE.

A GREENSTICK FRACTURE only occurs in young children whose bones are still soft and tend to bend. The fracture occurs on the opposite side from the causal force. A *complicated fracture* involves damage to surrounding soft tissue including nerves and blood vessels. A *depressed fracture* refers only to the skull when a piece of bone is forced inwards and may damage the brain. *See also* COMMINUTED FRACTURE.

Friedreich's ataxia an inherited disorder caused by degeneration of nerve cells in the brain and spinal cord. It appears in children, usually in adolescence, and the symptoms include unsteadiness during walking and a loss of the knee-jerk reflex, leading progressively to tremors, speech impairment and curvature of the spine. The symptoms are increasingly disabling and may be accompanied by heart disease. *See also* ATAXIA.

frontal lobe the anterior part of the *cerebral hemisphere* of the CEREBRUM of the brain, extending back to a region called the central sulcus which is a deep cleft on the upper, outer surface.

frostbite damage to the skin and underlying tissues caused by extreme cold and especially affecting the 'extremities' i.e. fingers, toes, nose and cheeks. The affected parts become white and numb and may develop blisters. The skin hardens and gradually turns black, and if the frostbite is fairly superficial, this eventually peels off exposing tender red skin underneath. However, in severe cases, deeper layers of tissue become frozen and are destroyed and amputation may be necessary especially where infection has set in. *See* GANGRENE.

frozen shoulder painful stiffness of the shoulder joint which limits movement and is more common in older people between the ages of 50 and 70. It may result from injury but often there is no apparent cause. Treatment involves exercises and sometimes injections of corticosteroid drugs, and usually there is a gradual recovery.

fundus the enlarged base of an organ farthest away from its opening or a point in the RETINA of the EYE opposite the pupil.

fungal diseases diseases or infections caused by fungi.

G

galactorrhoea flow of milk from the breast, not associated with childbirth or nursing. It may be a symptom of a tumour in the pituitary gland.

gall another term for BILE.

gall bladder a sac-like organ situated on the underside of the liver which stores and concentrates BILE. It is approximately 8cm long and 2.5cm at its widest and its volume is a little over 30cm³. When fats are digested, the gall bladder contracts, sending bile into the DUODENUM through the common bile duct. GALLSTONES, the most common gall bladder disease, may form in certain circumstances.

gallstones stones of varying composition, that form in the GALL BLADDER. Their formation seems to be due to a change in bile composition rendering cholesterol less soluble. Stones may also form around a foreign body. There are three types of stone: cholesterol, pigment and mixed, the latter being the most common. Calcium salts are usually found in vary-

ing proportions. Although gallstones may be present for years without symptoms, they can cause severe pain and may pass into the common bile duct to cause, by the resulting obstruction, jaundice.

gamete a mature germ or sexual cell, male or female, that can participate in fertilization e.g. OVUM and SPERMATOZOON.

gamma globulin (or immune gamma GLOBULIN) a concentrated form of the antibody part of human blood. It is used for immunization against certain infectious diseases, e.g. measles, poliomyelitis, hepatitis A, etc. It is of no use when the disease is diagnosed but can prevent or modify it if given before.

ganglion (*plural* **ganglia**) 1. a mass of nervous tissue containing nerve cells and SYNAPSES. Chains of ganglia are situated on each side of the spinal cord while other ganglia are sited near to or in the appropriate organs. Within the central nervous system some well-defined masses of nerve cells are called ganglia e.g. basal ganglia (*see* BASAL GANGLION).

2. a benign swelling that often forms in the sheath of a tendon and is fluid-filled. It occurs particularly at the wrist, and may disappear quite suddenly.

gangrene death of tissue due to loss of blood supply or bacterial infection. There are two types of gangrene, *dry* and *moist*. Dry gangrene is caused purely by loss of blood supply and is a late stage complication of DIABETES MELLITUS in which ATHEROSCLEROSIS is present. The affected part becomes cold and turns brown and black and there is an obvious line between living and dead tissue. In time the gangrenous part drops off.

Moist gangrene is the more common type and is due to bacterial infection which leads to putrefaction and issuing of fluids from the tissue, accompanied by an obnoxious smell. The patient may suffer from fever and ultimately die of blood poisoning. (*See also* GAS GANGRENE.)

gas gangrene a form of GANGRENE that occurs when wounds are infected with soil bacteria of the genus *Clostridium*. The bacterium produces toxins that cause decay and putrefaction with the generation of gas. The gas spreads into muscles and connective tissue causing swelling, pain, fever and possibly toxic delirium, and if untreated the condition quickly leads to death. Some of these bacteria are anaerobic (exist without air or oxygen) hence surgery, oxidizing agents and penicillin can all be used in treatment.

gastralgia term meaning pain in the stomach.

gastrectomy the surgical removal of, usually, part of the stomach. This may be performed for stomach cancer, severe peptic ulcers or to stop haemorrhaging.

gastric anything relating to the stomach.

gastric glands glands that are situated in the MUCOUS MEMBRANE of the stomach and secrete GASTRIC JUICE. The glands are the *cardiac, pyloric* and *fundic*.

gastric juice the secretion from the GASTRIC GLANDS in the stomach. The main constituents are hydrochloric acid, rennin, mucin and pepsinogen, the latter forming pepsin in the acid conditions. The acidity (which is around pH 1 to 1.5) also destroys unwanted bacteria.

gastric ulcer an erosion of the stomach MUCOSA caused by such agents as acid and bile. It may penetrate the muscle and perforate the stomach wall (*see* PERFORATION). Typical symptoms include burning pain, belching and possibly nausea when the stomach is empty or soon after eating. Relief may be found with antacid compounds, but surgery may be necessary.

gastritis inflammation of the stomach lining (MUCOSA). It may be due to bacteria or excessive alcohol intake.

gastroenteritis inflammation of both the stomach and intestines leading to vomiting, diarrhoea. It is most commonly due to viral or bacterial infection and fluid loss can be serious in children.

gastroenterology the study of diseases that affect the gastrointestinal tract including the pancreas, gall bladder and bile duct in addition to the stomach and intestines.

gastroenterostomy an operation undertaken to reroute food from the stomach to enable an obstruction to be relieved. It consists of making an opening in the stomach and the nearby small intestine and joining the two together. It is often performed with a gastrectomy.

gastroscope a flexible instrument comprising fibre optics or a miniature video camera that permits internal visual examination of the stomach. It is possible to see all areas of the stomach and take specimens using special tools. The tube is introduced via the mouth and oesophagus.

gastrostomy the creation, usually by surgery, of an opening into the stomach from the outside. This permits food to be given to a patient who cannot swallow due to oesophageal cancer, post-oesophageal surgery or who may be unconscious for a long time.

gauze a material with open weave that is used for bandages and dressings.

gavage forced feeding. Adopted when a patient is too weak to feed themselves or when an insane person refuses food. A stomach tube or naso-gastric tube is used.

gene the fundamental unit of genetic material found at a specific location on a CHROMOSOME. It is chemically complex and responsible for the transmission of information between older and younger generations. Each gene contributes to a particular trait or characteristic. There are more than 100,000 genes in man and gene size varies with the characteristic e.g. the

gene that codes for the hormone IN-SULIN is 1700 BASE PAIRS long.

There are several types of gene, depending upon their function and in addition genes are said to be dominant or recessive. A dominant characteristic is one that occurs whenever the gene is present while the effect of a recessive gene (say a disease) requires that the gene be on both members of the chromosome pair that is, it must be homozygous (*see also* SEX-LINKED DISORDERS).

genetic code specific information carried by DNA molecules that controls the particular AMINO ACIDS and their positions in every protein and thus all the proteins synthesized within a cell. Because there are just four nucleotides a unit of three bases becomes the smallest unit that can produce codes for all 20 amino acids. The transfer of information from gene to protein is based upon three consecutive nucleotides called *codons*. A change in the genetic code results in an amino acid being inserted incorrectly in a protein, resulting in a mutation.

genetic counselling the provision of advice to families about the nature and likelihood of inherited disorders and the options available in terms of prevention and management. With modern techniques of antenatal diagnosis it is possible to determine at an early stage of a pregnancy whether a child will be abnormal.

genetic engineering (or recombinant DNA technology) the artificial modification of an organism's genetic make-up. More specifically for example, the insertion of GENES from a human cell which are inserted into a bacterium where they perform their usual function. Thus it is possible to produce, on a commercial scale, hormones such as INSULIN and GROWTH HORMONE by utilizing a bacterium with a human gene. The organism often used is *Escherichia coli*. The process has other applications, including production of monoclonal antibodies.

genetic fingerprinting the technique that utilises an individual's DNA to identify that person. DNA can be extracted from body tissues and used in settling issues of a child's maternity or paternity. In forensic medicine samples of blood etc. at the scene of a crime are taken to match a suspect to the criminal.

genetics the study of heredity and variation in individuals and the means whereby characteristics are passed from parent to offspring. The classical aspects of the subject were expounded by Mendel, an Austrian monk, in the early 19th century. Now there are several subdisciplines, including population genetics and molecular genetics.

genetic screening the procedure whereby individuals are tested to determine whether their gene make-up suggests they carry a particular disease or condition. If it is shown that someone carries a genetically-linked disease then decisions can be taken regarding future children (*see also* SEX-LINKED DISORDERS).

genital the term describing anything relating to reproduction or the reproductive organs.

genitalia the male or female reproductive organs, often referring to the external parts only.

genito-urinary medicine the subdiscipline concerned with all aspects of sexually transmitted diseases.

genito-urinary tract (urogenital in US) the genital and urinary organs and associated structures: kidneys, ureter, bladder, urethra and genitalia.

geriatrics the subdiscipline of medicine that deals with all aspects of diseases and conditions that affected the aged.

german measles (*or* **rubella**) a highly infectious viral disease occurring mainly in childhood, but which is mild in effect. Spread occurs through close contact with infected individuals and there is an incubation period of two to three weeks. The symptoms include headache, shivering and sore throat with a slight fever. There is some swelling of the neck and soon after the onset a rash of pink spots appears, initially on the face and/or neck, and subsequently spreading over the body. The rash disappears in roughly one week but the condition remains infectious for 3 or 4 more days.

Immunity is usually conferred by the infection and although it is a mild disease it is important because an attack during the early stages of pregnancy may cause foetal abnormalities. Girls are therefore immunized around the age of 12 or 13.

germs microorganisms. The term is used particularly for microorganisms that are PATHOGENIC.

gestation the length of time from fertilization of the ovum to birth (*see also* PREGNANCY).

giddiness *see* VERTIGO.

gingivitis inflammation of the gums.

gland an organ or group of cells that

secretes a specific substance or substances. ENDOCRINE GLANDS secrete directly into the blood while *exocrine* glands secrete onto an epithelial surface via a duct. Some glands produce fluids, e.g. milk from the mammary glands, saliva from the sublingual bland and others. The THYROID gland is an endocrine gland releasing hormones into the bloodstream. A further system of glands, the lymphatic glands, occur throughout the body in association with the lymphatic vessels (*see* LYMPH).

glandular fever (*also known as* **infectious mononucleosis**) an infectious viral disease caused by the Epstein-Barr virus. It produces a sore throat and swelling in neck lymph nodes (also those in the armpits and groin). Other symptoms include headache, fever and a loss of appetite. The liver may be affected and the SPLEEN may become enlarged or even ruptured which then requires surgery. The disease is diagnosed by the large number of MONOCYTES in the blood and although complications tend to be rare, total recovery may take many weeks.

glaucoma a condition which results in loss of vision due to high pressure in the EYE, although there is usually no associated disease of the eye. There are several types of glaucoma which occur at differing rates but all are characterized by high intra-ocular pressure (due to the outflow of AQUEOUS HUMOUR being restricted) which damages nerve fibres in the RETINA and optic nerve. Treatment involves reduction of the pressure with drops and tablets (to reduce production of aqueous humour) and if necessary

surgery is undertaken to create another outlet for the aqueous humour.

gleet discharge due to chronic GONORRHOEA.

glia (**neuroglia** *or* **glial cells**) CENTRAL NERVOUS SYSTEM connective tissue composed of a variety of cells. The *macroglia* are divided into astrocytes that surround brain capillaries and oligodendrocytes that form MYELIN sheaths. The *microglia* perform a mainly scavenging function. Glial cells are present in ten to fifty times the number of neurons in the nervous system.

globulin a group of globular proteins that occur widely in milk, blood, eggs and plants. There are four types in blood SERUM: α_1, α_2, β, and γ. The alpha and beta types are carrier proteins like haemoglobin and gamma globulins include the IMMUNOGLOBULINS involved in the immune response.

glottis the opening between the VOCAL CHORDS. Also used for the part of the LARYNX involved with sound production.

glucagon a hormone important in maintaining the level of the body's blood sugar. It works antagonistically with INSULIN, increasing the supply of blood sugar through the breakdown of GLYCOGEN to glucose in the liver. Glucagon is produced by the ISLETS OF LANGERHANS when blood sugar level is low.

glue ear (*or* **secretory otitis media**) a form of OTITIS, common in children, which occurs as an inflammation of the middle ear with the production of a persistent sticky fluid. It can cause deafness and may be associated with enlarged adenoids. In treatment of the condition the adenoids may be removed and GROMMETs inserted.

gluteal the term given to the buttocks or the muscles forming them.

gluteus one of the three muscles of each buttock. The *gluteus maximus* shapes the buttock and extends the thigh, the *gluteus medius* and *minimus* abduct (move the limb away from the body) the thigh while the former also rotates it.

glycogen sometimes called animal starch, is a carbohydrate (polysaccharide) stored mainly in the liver. It acts as an energy store which is liberated upon hydrolysis (*see* GLUCAGON).

glycosuria the presence of sugar (glucose) in the urine which is usually due to DIABETES MELLITUS.

goitre swelling of the neck due to THYROID GLAND enlargement. The thyroid tries to counter the dietary lack of iodine necessary to produce thyroid hormone, by increasing the output, thereby becoming larger. The endemic or simple goitre is due to this cause. Other types are caused by HYPERPLASIA and autoimmune diseases, for example when antibodies are produced against antigens in the thyroid gland.

gold salts (or gold compound) chemicals containing gold that are used in minute quantities to treat RHEUMATOID ARTHRITIS. It is given by injection into muscles and because side effects may include skin reactions, blood disorders, mouth ulcers and inflammation of the kidneys, very careful control is kept on the dosage.

gonad the reproductive organs that produce the GAMETES and some hormones. In the male and female the gonads are the testes and ovaries respectively.

gonadotrophin (*or* **gonadotrophic hormone**) hormones secreted by the anterior PITUITARY GLAND. Folliclestimulating hormone (FSH) is produced by males and females as is luteinizing hormone, LH, (interstitial cell-stimulating hormone, ICSH, in males). FSH controls, directly or indirectly, growth of the ova and sperm, while LH/ICSH stimulates reproductive activity in the GONADS.

gonorrhoea the most common VENEREAL DISEASE which is spread primarily by sexual intercourse but may be contracted through contact with infected discharge on clothing, towels etc. The causative agent is the bacterium *Neisseria gonorrhoeae* and it affects the mucous membrane of the vagina, or in the male, the urethra. Symptoms develop approximately one week after infection and include pain on urinating with a discharge of pus. Inflammation of nearby organs may occur (testicle, prostate in men; uterus, Fallopian tubes and ovaries in women) and prolonged inflammation of the urethra may lead to formation of fibrous tissue causing STRICTURE. Joints may also be affected and later complications include ENDOCARDITIS, arthritis and CONJUNCTIVITIS.

If a baby is born to a woman with the disease, the baby's eyes may become infected, until recently a major cause of blindness (called *ophthalmia neonatorum*). Treatment is usually very effective through the administration of penicillin, sulphonamides or tetracycline.

gout a disorder caused by an imbalance of URIC ACID in the body. Uric acid is normally excreted by the kidneys but sufferers of gout have an excess in their bloodstream which is deposited in joints as salts (urates) of the acid. This causes inflammation of the affected joints and painful gouty arthritis with destruction of the joints. The kidneys may also be damaged, with formation of stones. Deposits of the salts (called *tophi*) may reach the stage where they prohibit further use of the joints, causing hands and feet to be set in a particular position. Treatment of gout is through drugs that increase the excretion of the urate salts or slow their formation.

Graafian follicle *see* FOLLICLE.

graft the removal of some tissue or an organ from one person for application to or implantation into the same person or another individual. For example, a skin graft involves taking healthy skin from one area of the body to heal damaged skin, and a kidney (or renal) graft (or transplant) is the removal of the organ from one person (usually a recently dead individual) to another. Numerous types of graft are now feasible, including skin, bone, cornea, cartilage, nerves and blood vessels, and whole organs such as kidney, heart and lung.

Gram's stain a technique described by H.C.J. Gram, the Danish bacteriologist in 1884, which involves using a stain to differentiate between certain bacteria. Bacteria on a microscope slide are first stained with a violet dye and iodine, then rinsed in ethanol to decolour and a second red stain added. *Gram-positive* bacteria keep the first stain and appear violet when examined under the micro-

scope, while *Gram-negative* forms lose the first but take up the second stain, thus appearing red. The difference in staining is due to the structure of the bacteria cell walls.

grand mal a convulsive epileptic fit involving involuntary muscular contractions and lack of respiration. The latter produces bluish skin and lips (CYANOSIS) during the *tonic* phase. Convulsive movements follow and often the tongue is bitten and bladder control is lost (the *clonic* phase). Upon awakening the patient has no recall of the event.

Grave's disease a disorder typified by thyroid gland overactivity (*see* HYPERTHYROIDISM), an enlargement of the gland, and protruding eyes. It is due to antibody production and is probably an autoimmune response (*see* AUTOIMMUNE DISEASE). Patients commonly exhibit excess metabolism (because thyroid hormones control the body's metabolism); nervousness, tremor, hyperactivity, rapid heart rate, an intolerance of heat, breathlessness and so on. Treatment may follow one of three courses; drugs to control the thyroid's production of hormones; surgery to remove part of the thyroid; or radioactive iodine therapy.

gravid another term for pregnant.

greenstick fracture *see* FRACTURE.

grey matter a part of the CENTRAL NERVOUS SYSTEM comprising the central part of the spinal cord and the cerebral cortex and outer layer of the cerebellum in the brain. It is brown-grey in colour and is the coordination point between the nerves of the central nervous system. It is composed of nerve cell bodies, DENDRITES,

SYNAPSES, glial cells (supporting cells, *see* GLIA) and blood vessels.

groin the areas where the abdomen joins the thighs.

grommet a small tube with a lip at either end that is inserted into the eardrum to permit fluid to drain from the middle ear. It is used in the treatment of secretory otitis media (GLUE EAR).

growing pains pains similar to rheumatism that occur in the joints and muscles of children. They are usually insignificant and may be due to fatigue or bad posture but must be dealt with in case the cause is more serious e.g. bone disease, or rheumatic fever.

growth hormone (somatotrophin or FH) a HORMONE produced and stored by the anterior PITUITARY GLAND that controls protein synthesis in muscles and the growth of long bones in legs and arms. Low levels result in DWARFISM in children and overproduction produces gigantism.

gullet another term for the OESOPHAGUS.

gynaecology the subdiscipline of medicine that deals with diseases of women, particularly concerning sexual and reproduction function and diseases of reproductive organs.

H

haem a compound containing iron, composed of a pigment which is known as a *porphyrin* which confers colour. It combines with a protein called globin in the blood to form HAEMOGLOBIN. The prefix *haem* also indicates anything relating to blood.

haemangioma a benign tumour of the blood vessels. It may be visible on the skin as a type of NAEVUS (birthmark) e.g. a *strawberry haemangioma*.

haemarthrosis bleeding into a joint which causes swelling and pain and may be the result of injury or disease. It can be a symptom of HAEMOPHILIA.

haematemesis vomiting of blood which may occur for a number of different reasons. Common causes

are ulcers, either gastric or duodenal, or gastritis, especially when this is caused by irritants or poisons such as alcohol. Also blood may be swallowed and subsequently vomited as a result of a nosebleed.

haematinic a substance which increases the amount of haemoglobin in the blood e.g. ferrous sulphate. Haematinic drugs are often prescribed during pregnancy.

haematocoele leakage of blood into a cavity causing a swelling. A haematocoele usually forms as a result of an injury due to the rupture of blood vessels and the leaking of blood into a natural body cavity.

haematology the scientific study of blood and its diseases.

haematoma a collection of blood forming a firm swelling-a bruise. It may occur as a result of injury, a clotting disorder of the blood or if blood vessels are diseased.

haematuria the presence of blood in the urine which may have come from the kidneys, ureters, bladder or urethra. It indicates the presence of inflammation or disease such as a stone in the bladder or kidney.

haemodialysis the use of an *artificial kidney* to remove waste products from a person's blood using the principle of DIALYSIS. It is carried out when a person's kidneys have ceased to function and involves passing blood from an artery into the dialyser on one side of a semipermeable membrane. On the other side of the membrane, a solution of electrolytes of similar composition to the blood is circulated. Water and waste products pass through the membrane into this solution while cells and proteins are retained within the blood. The purified blood is then returned to the patient's body through a vein.

haemoglobin the respiratory substance contained within the red blood cells which contains a pigment responsible for the red colour of blood. It consists of the pigment HAEM and the protein globin and is responsible for the transport of oxygen around the body. Oxygen is picked up in the lungs by arterial blood and transported to the tissues where it is released. This (venous) blood is then returned to the lungs to repeat the process (*see* OXYHAEMO-GLOBIN).

haemoglobinopathy any of a number of inherited diseases in which there is an abnormality in the formation of haemoglobin. Examples are thalassaemia and SICKLE CELL ANAEMIA.

haemoglobinuria the presence of haemoglobin in the urine caused by disintegration of red blood cells, conferring a dark red or brown colour. It can sometimes result from strenuous exercise or after exposure to cold in some people. It is also caused by the ingestion of poisons such as arsenic, and is a symptom of some infections, particularly *blackwater fever*, a severe and sometimes fatal form of MALARIA.

haemolysis the destruction (LYSIS) of red blood cells which may result from infection, poisoning or as an antibody response.

haemolytic disease of the newborn a serious disease affecting foetuses and newborn babies which is characterized by HAEMOLYSIS leading to anaemia and severe jaundice. In severe cases the foetus may die due to heart failure and OEDEMA (termed *hydrops foetalis*). The usual cause is incompatibility between the blood of the mother and that of the foetus. Generally the foetus has Rh positive red blood cells (i.e. they contain the rhesus factor) while that of the mother is Rh negative. The mother produces antibodies to the Rh factor present in the foetal blood and these are passed to the foetus in the placental circulation. This then produces the haemolysis of the foetal red blood cells.

The incidence of the disease has been greatly reduced by giving a Rh negative mother an injection of anti-D immunoglobulin, following the birth of a Rh positive baby. This prevents the formation of the antibodies which would harm a subsequent baby and is also given to Rh negative women following miscarriages or abortions.

haemophilia an hereditary disorder of blood coagulation in which the blood clots very slowly. It is a sex-linked recessive condition carried on the X chromosome and hence it affects males with females being the carriers. There are two types of haemophilia due to a deficiency of either one of two COAGULATION FACTORS in the blood. Haemophilia A is caused by deficiency of factor VIII and haemophilia B by deficiency of factor IX, called *Christmas factor*. The severity of the disease depends upon how much less of the coagulation factor than normal is present in the blood. The symptoms of haemophilia are prolonged bleeding from wounds and bleeding into joints, muscles and other tissues. In the past, the outlook for haemophiliacs was poor with few surviving into adult life. However, now the condition can be treated by injections or transfusions of plasma containing the missing coagulation factor and, with care, a sufferer can hope to lead a much more normal life. *See* SEX-LINKED DISORDERS.

haemopoiesis formation of blood cells (particularly *erythrocytes*, the red blood cells) and platelets, which takes place in the bone marrow in adults but in a foetus it occurs in the liver and spleen.

haemorrhage bleeding - a flow of blood from a ruptured blood vessel which may occur externally or internally. A haemorrhage is classified according to the type of vessels involved: *Arterial H* - bright red blood spurts in pulses from an artery. *Venous H* - a darker coloured steady flow from a vein. *Capillary L* - blood oozes from torn capillaries at the surface of a wound. In addition, a haemorrhage may be *primary* i.e. it occurs at the moment of injury. It is classed as *reactionary* when it occurs within 24 hours of an injury and results from a rise in blood pressure. Thirdly, a *secondary haemorrhage* occurs after a week or ten days as a result of infection (sepsis). Haemorrhage from a major artery is the most serious kind as large quantities of blood are quickly lost and death can occur within minutes. Haemorrhages at specific sites within the body are designated by special names e.g. *haematuria* (from the kidney or urinary tract), *haemoptysis* (from the lungs) and *haematemesis* (from the stomach).

haemorrhoids (piles) varicose and inflamed veins around the lower end of the bowel situated in the wall of the anus. They are classified as internal, external and mixed depending upon whether they appear beyond the anus. They are commonly caused by constipation or diarrhoea, especially in middle and older age, and may be exacerbated by a sedentary life style. They may also occur as a result of childbearing. Symptoms of haemorrhoids are bleeding and pain, and treatment is by means of creams, injections and suppositories. Attention to diet (to treat constipation) and regular exercise are important, but in severe cases, surgery to remove the haemorrhoids may be necessary.

haemostasis the natural process to arrest bleeding involving blood coagulation and contraction of a ruptured blood vessel. The term is also applied to a number of surgical procedures designed to arrest bleeding such as the use of ligatures and DIATHERMY. A haemostatic substance stops or prevents haemorrhage e.g. phytomenadone.

haemothorax a leakage of blood into the pleural cavity of the chest, usually as a result of injury.

hair a threadlike outgrowth from the epidermis layer of the skin which is a dead structure consisting of KERATINIZED cells. The part above the skin has three layers, an outer CUTICLE, a CORTEX containing pigment which confers colour, and an inner core. The lower end of the hair (*root*) lies within the skin and is expanded to form the *bulb* which contains dividing cells that are continuously pushed upwards. This is contained within a tubular structure known as the *hair follicle*. A small *erector pili* muscle attached to the hair follicle in the DERMIS of the skin operates to erect the hair.

halitosis 'bad breath' which may arise for a number of reasons, including the type of food recently eaten, disease of the teeth or infections of the throat, nose and lungs.

hallucination a false perception of something that is not there and which may involve any of the senses of sight, hearing, smell, taste and touch. They may be caused by a psychological illness e.g. SCHIZOPHRENIA or damage to the brain, and also by certain drugs. They can also be a symptom of fever and deprivation such as lack of sleep.

hallucinogen a substance or drug which causes HALLUCINATIONS e.g. mescaline and lysergic acid diethylamide.

hammer toe *see* CORN.

hamstring any of four tendons at the back of the knee which are attached to the *hamstring muscles* and anchor these to the TIBIA and FIBULA. The hamstring muscles are responsible for the bending of the knee joint.

hand the extremity of the upper limb below the wrist which has a highly complex structure and an 'opposable' thumb which is unique to man. The human hand is highly developed in terms of structure, nervous supply and function and communicates with a large area on the surface of the brain. It is capable of performing numerous functions with a high degree of precision. When there is brain damage and paralysis, the uses of the hand tend to be lost early and more permanently compared to movements in the leg and face. The skeletal structure of the hand consists of eight small *carpal* bones in the wrist, five *metacarpal* bones in the region of the palm and three *phalanges* in each finger.

haploid the description for a cell nucleus or organism with half the normal number of chromosomes. This is the case with GAMETES and is important at fertilization to ensure the *diploid* chromosome number is restored.

hare lip a congenital developmental deformity which results in the presence of a cleft in the upper lip. It is brought about by a failure in the fusion of three blocks of embryonic tissue and is often associated with a CLEFT PALATE.

Hartmann's solution a solution of salts which is given to replace lost fluid in cases of dehydration, acidosis and after HAEMORRHAGE while awaiting cross-matched blood for transfusion.

Haversian canal one of numerous small channels or cylindrical tubes which run through compact bone (the outer layer of bones) and contain blood vessels and nerves. They form part of the *Haversian system* consisting of the canals surrounded by concentric, alternate layers of bone *lamellae* and *lacunae* or spaces, which house bone cells. These form cylindrical units in the compact bone and the lacunae are linked up by minute channels called *caniculi*.

hay fever an allergic reaction to pollen e.g. that of grasses, trees and many other plants which affects numerous individuals. The symptoms are a blocked and runny nose, sneezing and watering eyes due to the release of histamine. Treatment is by means of antihistamine drugs and, if the allergen can be identified, *desensitization* may be successful. This involves injecting or exposing the individual to controlled and gradually increasing doses of the allergen until antibodies are built up.

headache pain felt within the head which is thought to be caused by dilation of intracranial arteries or pressure upon them. Common causes are stress, tiredness, feverishness accompanying an infection such as a cold, an excess of close work involving the eyes, dyspepsia, rheumatic diseases, high blood pressure and uraemia. Headache may indicate the presence of disease or disorder in the brain e.g. an infection such as MENINGITIS, TUMOUR or ANEURYSM and also as a result of injury and concussion.

heart the hollow, muscular organ which acts as a pump and is responsible for the circulation of the blood. The heart is cone-shaped with the point downwards and is situated between the lungs and slightly to the left of the midline. The heart projects forwards and lies beneath the fifth rib. The wall consists mainly of CARDIAC MUSCLE lined on the inside by a membrane known as the ENDOCARDIUM. An external membrane known as the PERICARDIUM surrounds the heart. A SEPTUM divides the heart into right and left halves, each of which is further divided into an upper chamber known as an ATRIUM and a lower one called a VENTRICLE. Four valves control the direction of blood flow at each outlet, comprising the aortic, pulmonary, tricuspid and mitral (bicuspid). These valves prevent backflow once the blood has been forced from one chamber into the next. *See* CIRCULATION OF THE BLOOD.

heart attack *see* CARDIAC ARREST.

heart block a condition describing a failure in the conduction of electrical impulses from the natural pacemaker (the SINOATRIAL NODE) through the heart, which can lead to slowing of the pumping action.

There are three types: in first degree (partial or incomplete) heart block there is a delay in conduction between atria (*see* ATRIUM) and VEN-

TRICLES but this does not cause slowing. In second degree heart block, there is intermittent slowing because not all the impulses are conducted between atria and ventricles. In third degree (or complete) heart block there is no electrical conduction, the heartbeats are slow and the ventricles beat at their own intrinsic slow rhythm. This causes blackouts (known as Stokes-Adams syndrome) and can lead to heart failure.

Heart block is more common in elderly people where degenerative changes have occurred. However, it may also be CONGENITAL or result from other forms of heart disease such as MYOCARDITIS, CORONARY THROMBOSIS, CARDIOMYOPATHY and VALVE DISEASE. For second and third degree heart block, treatment involves the use of an artificial pacemaker.

heartburn a burning pain or discomfort felt in the region of the heart and often rising upwards to the throat. It is caused by regurgitation of the stomach contents, the burning being caused by the acid in gastric juice or by OESOPHAGITIS. It is relieved by taking antacid tablets or alkaline substances such as sodium bicarbonate.

heat exhaustion exhaustion and collapse due to overheating of the body and loss of fluid following unaccustomed or prolonged exposure to excessive heat. It is more common in hot climates and results from excessive sweating leading to loss of fluids and salts and disturbance of the electrolyte balance in body fluids. In the mildest form which is *heat collapse*, blood pressure and pulse rate fall accompanied by fatigue, light-headedness and there may be muscular cramps.

heat stroke or **heat hyperpyrexia** a severe condition following exposure of the body to excessive heat characterized by a rise in temperature and failure of sweating and temperature regulation. There is a loss of consciousness, followed by coma and death which can occur rapidly. The body must be cooled by sponging and salt solutions given either by mouth or intravenously.

heel the part of the foot behind the ankle joint formed by the *calcaneus* or heel bone.

Heimlich's manoeuvre a procedure to dislodge a foreign body which is blocking the larynx causing CHOKING. The person carrying out the procedure encircles the patient from behind with his arms. A fist is made with one hand slightly above the patient's navel and below the ribs. With the free hand, the fist is thrust firmly into the abdomen with a rapid upward push which may need to be repeated several times. As a result of this, the foreign particle is expelled through or into the patient's mouth.

Henle's loop *see* KIDNEY.

heparin an anticoagulant substance naturally present in the body, and produced by liver and some white blood cells and in some other sites. It acts by inhibiting and neutralizing the action of the enzyme thrombin (*see* BLOOD COAGULATION) and is a polysaccharide (carbohydrate) containing sulphur and amino groups. It is used medically to prevent blood coagulation in patients with thrombosis and also in blood collected for sampling.

hepatectomy surgical removal of the whole or part of the liver.

hepatic vein one of the veins which drains blood from the liver leading to the inferior vena cava.

hepatitis inflammation of the liver due to the presence of toxic substances or infection caused by viruses. *Acute hepatitis* produces abdominal pain, jaundice, itching, nausea and fever. *Chronic hepatitis* has a similar range of symptoms which may persist for years and lead eventually to CIRRHOSIS. Alcohol abuse is a common cause of hepatitis which may also result as a side effect from a number of drug treatments or from overdose. Many virus infections can cause hepatitis such as HIV and GLANDULAR FEVER.

However, the so-called hepatic viruses are designated A, B, C, D, and E. Hepatitis A causes *infectious hepatitis* (epidemic hepatitis) and is transmitted by eating food contaminated by a person who has the virus, and is common in conditions of poor hygiene and sanitation. Hepatitis E acts in a similar way and both produce symptoms of fever, sickness and jaundice. Recovery is usually complete unless the symptoms are acute and immunity from a future attack is conferred. *Serum hepatitis* is caused by viruses B, C and D, the route of infection being blood or blood products. Serum hepatitis is most common where infected needles have been used among drug addicts. The infection may also be passed on by tattooing needles and also through sexual intercourse with an infected individual. The mortality rate is 5 - 20%, but many patients make a gradual recovery from the illness which is characterized by fever, chills, fatigue, headaches and jaundice. All these viruses may persist in the blood for a long time and if B is involved, the condition is known as *chronic type - B hepatitis*. Cancer (hepatocellular carcinoma) is common in populations where the B virus is prevalent. Various drugs are used to combat viral hepatitis including interferon.

hepatoma a malignant tumour of the liver which is rare in Western countries except among those with CIRRHOSIS. It is common in parts of the Far East and Africa and a suspected cause is the *aflatoxin* or poison produced by a fungus which contaminates stored peanuts and cereals. The cancer often produces alpha fetoprotein which is detectable in the blood and is an indicator of the presence of the malignancy.

heredity the principle applied to the passing on of all bodily characteristic from parents to offspring. *See* GENETICS.

hermaphrodite an individual possessing both male and female sex organs or in whom ovarian and testicular cells are present in the gonads (*ovotestis*). This condition is extremely rare and the individual is usually sterile with reduced SECONDARY SEXUAL CHARACTERISTICS.

hernia the protrusion of a part or whole of an organ from out of its normal position within the body cavity. Most commonly, a hernia involves part of the bowel. A *congenital hernia* is present at birth, a common one being an *umbilical hernia* in which abdominal organs protrude into the umbilical cord. This is due to a failure during foetal development and can be corrected by surgery. An *acquired hernia* occurs after birth, a common example being an *inguinal hernia* in which part of the bowel bulges through a weak part of the abdominal wall, (known as the inguinal canal). Another common type is a *hiatus hernia* in which the stomach passes through the hiatus (a hole allowing passage of the oesophagus), from the abdomen into the chest cavity. A *reducible hernia* is freely movable and can be returned by manipulation into its rightful place. An *irreducible hernia* describes the opposite situation and an *incarcerated hernia* is one which has become swollen and fixed in its position. An *obstructed hernia* is one involving the bowel. The contents of the hernia are unable to pass further down and are held up and obstructed.

The most dangerous situation is a *strangulated hernia* in which the blood supply has been cut off due to the protrusion itself. This becomes painful and eventually gangrenous and requires immediate surgery as it is life-threatening. Strenuous physical activity can lead to the production of a hernia which usually develops gradually. Although short-term measures are employed to control a hernia or reduce its size, the usual treatment is by means of surgery to return and retain the protrusion in its proper place. *See* HERNIOPLASTY.

hernioplasty the surgical operation to repair a hernia.

heroin a white crystalline powder, also known as dimorphine hydrochloride, which is derived from mor-

phine. It is a very potent analgesic (painkiller), but is highly addictive and dangerous.

herpes infectious inflammation of the skin and mucous membranes, characterized by the development of small blisters, and caused by a number of different *Herpes viruses*. The *Herpes simplex* virus, types I and II, are the cause of cold sores which usually affect the lips, mouth and face. The virus is usually acquired in childhood and once present persists for life. It can be contracted without causing any symptoms but tends to flare up from time to time producing the cold sores.

Herpes simplex is also the cause of genital herpes in which the blisters affect the genital region. *Herpes zoster* or shingles is produced by a virus which causes chicken pox in children. The virus affects the course of a nerve producing severe pain and small yellowish blisters on the skin. Often the affected areas are the abdomen, back, face and chest and although the disease subsides after about three weeks, the blisters form scabs which eventually drop off and the pain can persist for months. This is known as *post-herpetic neuralgia* and pain-relieving drugs are needed to help relieve the condition. Other Herpes viruses are the cytomegalovirus and EPSTEIN BARR virus.

hiatus hernia *see* HERNIA.

hindbrain the part of the brain which consists of the MEDULLA OBLONGATA, PONS and CEREBELLUM.

hip the region on either side of the body where the FEMUR (thigh bone) articulates with the PELVIS.

hip joint a *'ball and socket'* joint

made up of the head of the FEMUR which rests inside a deep, cup-shaped cavity (the acetabulum), in the hip bone. The hip bone (or innominate bone) is itself made up of three fused bones, the PUBIS, ISCHIUM and ILIUM which form part of the PELVIS.

hirsutism the growth of dark, coarse hair on the body of a female on the face, chest, abdomen and upper back. This is either due to a greater sensitivity of hair follicles to a normal level of male hormones (androgens) producing hair of a more masculine type. Or, there may be an excessive production of androgens responsible for the growth of the hair. The condition may be the result of an underlying disorder such as an ADRENAL tumour but there is a wide normal variation in the amount of body hair present in individuals and between females of different races.

histamine a substance derived from histidine which is an amino acid. It is widely found throughout all the body tissues and is responsible for the dilation of blood vessels (arterioles and capillaries) and the contraction of smooth muscle, including that of the bronchi of the lungs. Histamine is released in great quantities in allergic conditions and ANAPHYLAXIS (*see also* ALLERGY).

histology the scientific study of tissues, involving such techniques as light and electron microscopy and the use of dyes and stains.

HIV the human immunodeficiency virus responsible for the condition known as AIDS. The virus affects and destroys a group of lymphocytes (T-lymphocytes) which are part of the body's natural defences (the IMMUNE SYSTEM).

hives a common name for urticaria or nettle rash.

Hodgkin's disease a malignant disease of unknown cause affecting the lymphatic system in which there is a gradual and increasing enlargement of lymph glands and nodes throughout the body. The accompanying symptoms include loss of weight, sweating, anaemia and a characteristic type of fever (known as Pel-Ebstein fever). The person becomes gradually weaker and the glands may attain a very large size. The outlook is good, especially if the disease is detected early.

holistic relating to 'wholeness.' A holistic approach to patient care does not just concentrate on the physical disease or condition but takes note of all the factors in that person's life.

homeopathy a system of medicine devised by Samuel Hahnemann (1755 - 1843) which is a form of ALTERNATIVE MEDICINE in the U.K. It is based on the premise that 'like cures like' and so a patient is given minute quantities of drugs that can, in themselves, produce symptoms of the disease or malady being treated.

HRT *see* MENOPAUSE.

hormone a naturally-produced chemical substance produced by the body which acts as a messenger. A hormone is produced by cells or glands in one part of the body and passes into the bloodstream. When it reaches another specific site, its 'target organ,' it causes a reaction there, modifying the structure or function of cells, perhaps by causing the release of another hormone. Hormones are secreted by the ENDOCRINE GLANDS and examples are the sex hormones, e.g. TESTOSTERONE secreted by the testes and oestradiol and PROGESTERONE secreted by the ovaries.

housemaid's knee a painful condition resulting from a swelling of the bursa (fluid-filled fibrous sac) in front of the kneecap.

human chorionic gonadotrophin a hormone secreted by the PLACENTA during early pregnancy under the influence of which the CORPUS LUTEUM of the OVARY produces OESTROGEN, PROGESTERONE and relaxin. These are essential for the maintenance of pregnancy. Pregnancy can be detected early on by a laboratory procedure which tests for the presence of human chorionic gonadotrophin in the urine.

human T-cell lymphocytotrophic virus (HTLV) a group of viruses including the AIDS (HIV) virus which is HTLV III. These viruses are responsible for LYMPHOMAS.

humerus the bone of the upper arm which articulates with the shoulder blade (SCAPULA) of the PECTORAL GIRDLE and the ULNA and RADIUS at the elbow.

humour a natural fluid in the body, the best known examples being the aqueous and vitreous humours of the EYE.

Huntington's chorea *see* **chorea**.

hydrocephalus an abnormal collection of cerebrospinal fluid within the skull which causes, in babies and children, a great increase in the size of the head. Hydrocephalus results either from an excessive production of fluid or from a defect in the mechanism for its reabsorption, or from a blockage in its circulation.

The cause may be CONGENITAL, and it often accompanies SPINA BIFIDA in babies, or infection (meningitis) or the presence of a TUMOUR. Hydrocephalus causes pressure on the brain with drowsiness, irritability and mental subnormality in children. Treatment involves surgery to redirect the fluid but is not always successful. About 50% of children survive if the progress of the condition is halted and one third of these go on to enjoy a normal life with little or no physical or mental impairment.

hydrocortisone a STEROID glucocorticoid hormone, produced and released by the cortex of the ADRENAL GLANDS (a CORTICOSTEROID). It is closely related to cortisone being released in response to stress and playing a significant part in carbohydrate metabolism. Medically it has a number of uses especially in the treatment of ADDISON'S DISEASE, inflammatory, allergic and rheumatic conditions e.g. eczema and rheumatoid arthritis. Hydrocortisone is contained in ointments in creams or given by mouth or injection depending upon the condition under treatment. Prolonged use may cause side effects including peptic ulcers, stunting of growth in children, CUSHING'S SYNDROME and damage to bone and muscle tissue.

hydroxocobalamin this is a cobalt-containing (cobalamin) substance used in the treatment of vitamin B_{12} deficiencies, such as pernicious ANAEMIA.

hymen a thin membrane that covers the lower end of the VAGINA at birth which usually tears to some extent before a girl reaches puberty.

hyperadrenalism a condition in which the adrenal glands are overactive producing the symptoms of CUSHING'S SYNDROME.

hyperalgesia an extreme sensitivity to pain.

hyperglycaemia the presence of excess sugar (glucose) in the blood, as in DIABETES MELLITUS caused by insufficient INSULIN to cope with carbohydrate intake. The condition can lead to a diabetic coma.

hyperlipidaemia (hyperlipaemia) the presence of an excess concentration of fat in the blood. An excess of CHOLESTEROL in the blood may lead to CORONARY ARTERY DISEASE and ATHEROMA. An excess of triglycerides may lead to pancreatitis.

hyperplasia increased growth in size and number of the normal cells of a tissue so that the affected part enlarges e.g. the breasts during pregnancy. *Compare* HYPERTROPHY and NEOPLASM.

hypersensitivity abnormal allergic response to an ANTIGEN to which the person has previously been exposed. Hypersensitive responses vary from quite mild such as hay fever to very severe and life-threatening e.g. ANAPHYLACTIC SHOCK *(see also* ALLERGY).

hypertension high blood pressure (in the arteries). *Essential* hypertension is high blood pressure with no identifiable cause, or kidney disease or endocrine diseases. *Malignant* hypertension will prove fatal if not treated. It may be a condition itself or an end stage of essential hypertension. It tends to occur in a younger age group and there is high diastolic blood pressure *(see* DIASTOLE) and kidney failure.

Arteriosclerosis is a complication of, and often associated with hypertension. Other complications include cerebral haemorrhage, heart failure and kidney failure. Previously a rapidly fatal condition, antihypertensive drugs have revolutionized treatment and given sufferers a near-normal life. *See also* PULMONARY HYPERTENSION.

hyperthermia extremely high and abnormal body temperature i.e. a fever. Also, a method of treatment of certain diseases by artificially inducing a state of fever achieved by a variety of techniques.

hyperthyroidism excessive activity of the thyroid gland - an overactive thyroid. It may be caused by increased growth of the gland, by the presence of a tumour or due to GRAVES DISEASE.

hypertrophy increase in size of an organ due to enlargement of its cells (rather than in their number) often in response to a greater demand for work. An example is the increase in size of the remaining kidney if the other is removed for some reason. *Compare* HYPERPLASIA.

hyperventilation breathing at an abnormally rapid rate when at rest, which may be a response to stress and, if not checked, results in unconsciousness because the concentration of carbon dioxide in the blood falls. If the carbon dioxide level in the blood is abnormally high, due to impaired gas exchange in the lungs, e.g. in pulmonary OEDEMA and pneumonia, hyperventilation may occur. (*See also* HYPOVENTILATION.)

hypnotics substances or drugs that induce sleep e.g. BARBITURATES and *chloral hydrate*.

hypnosis a state of altered attention resembling sleep in which the mind is more receptive to recall of memories of past events and to suggestion. The person who induces this state in another is known as a *hypnotist*. One of the ways of inducing hypnosis is to ask the patient to fix his eyes on a given point or source of light and then rhythmically repeat soothing words in a low voice. Some people appear to be more easily *hypnotized* than others and there are three merging levels of hypnosis, *light, medium* and *deep*. Hypnosis is a useful form of treatment in psychiatry and also in pain relief e.g. during labour and dental repair. It is also used in the treatment of asthma and alcoholism.

hypochondria an abnormal preoccupation by an individual with the state of his or her health. In its severest form the person wrongly believes that he or she is suffering from a number of illnesses and is extremely anxious and depressed. Treatment is by means of psychotherapy and anti-depressant drugs but the condition tends to be difficult to cure.

hypodermic beneath the skin. The term is usually used in reference to injections given by means of a *hypodermic syringe*.

hypoglycaemia a lack of sugar in the blood which occurs in starvation and also with DIABETES MELLITUS when too much insulin has been given and insufficient carbohydrates have been eaten. The symptoms include weakness, sweating, light-headedness and tremors and can lead to coma. The symptoms are alleviated by taking in glucose either by mouth, or injection in the case of hypoglycaemic coma.

hypoplasia underdevelopment of a tissue or organ such as can occur in the teeth due to illness or starvation (dental hypoplasia). It is marked by lines across the teeth of brown enamel.

hypothalamus an area of the forebrain in the floor of the third ventricle, having the thalamus above and pituitary gland below. It contains centres controlling vital processes, e.g. fat and carbohydrate metabolism, thirst and water regulation, hunger and eating, thermal regulation and sexual function. It also plays a part in the emotions and in the regulation of sleep. It controls the sympathetic and parasympathetic nervous systems and secretions from the pituitary gland.

hypothermia describes the bodily state when the core temperature falls below 35°C due to prolonged exposure to cold. At first, shivering occurs and the heart works harder to increase the flow of blood around the body. However, eventually shivering ceases and, with increasing chilling, the function of the body organs becomes disturbed and cardiac output falls. The tissues require less oxygen as their functions start to fail, but eventually the heart is unable to supply even this reduced demand. The symptoms of hypothermia are fatigue and confusion followed by unconsciousness and death. Elderly people are particularly at risk through inadequate heating in the home.

Occasionally, a state of artificial hypothermia is induced during surgery to reduce the oxygen requirements of the tissues and enable the circulation to be briefly halted.

hypoventilation an abnormally slow rate of shallow breathing which may result from injury or the effects of drugs on the respiratory centre in the brain. The effect is to increase the amount of carbon dioxide in the blood and lessen that of oxygen. Eventually this leads to death due to a lack of oxygen supply to cells and tissues.

hysterectomy the surgical removal of the womb either by means of an abdominal incision or through the VAGINA. It is commonly carried out if fibroids are present or if the womb is cancerous, and also if there is excessive bleeding.

I

ichthyosis a generally hereditary skin condition in which the skin is very dry and looks cracked producing a resemblance to fish scales. There is particular medication to take but vitamin A may help. The treatment is thus external and involves special baths and the application of ointments.

idiopathic the term given to a disease indicating that its cause is not known.

ileitis inflammation of the ILEUM with pain, bowel irregularity and loss of weight. The intestine may become thickened and if the tract becomes blocked, surgery is required immediately. The specific cause is not known but it may occur in association with tuberculosis, bacterial infection (by *Yersinia enterocolitica*), Crohn's disease (chronic inflammation of the bowel) and typhoid.

ileectomy removal by surgery of all or part of the ILEUM.

ileostomy a surgical procedure in which an opening is made in the abdominal wall, to which the ileum is joined. This creates an artificial anus through which the waste contents of the intestines are collected in a special bag. This procedure is undertaken to allow the COLON to heal after surgery or colitis, or in association with other surgery in treating cancer of the rectum.

ileum the lower part of the small intestine between the JEJUNUM and the CAECUM.

ileus an obstruction of the intestine (often the ILEUM) which may be mechanical due to worms or a gallstone from the gall bladder, or it can be due to loss of the natural movement of the intestines (peristalsis). This latter condition may be caused by surgery, injury to the spine or PERITONITIS.

iliac arteries those arteries supplying blood to the lower limbs and pelvic region.

ilium the largest of the bones that form each half of the pelvic girdle. It has a flattened wing-like part fastening to the SACRUM by means of ligaments.

immune the state of being protected against an infection by the presence of antibodies specific to the organism concerned.

immunity the way in which the body resists infection due to the presence of ANTIBODIES and white blood cells. Antibodies are generated in response to the presence of ANTIGENS of a disease. There are several types of immunity: *active immunity* is when the body produces antibodies and continues to be able to do so, during the course of a disease whether occurring naturally (also called *acquired immunity*) or by deliberate stimulation. *Passive immunity* is short-lived and due to the injection of ready-made antibodies from someone who is already immune.

immunization producing immunity to disease by artificial means. Injection of an antiserum will produce temporary passive immunity. Active immunity is produced by making the body generate its own antibodies and this is done by the use of treated antigens (vaccination or INOCULATION). VACCINE is used for immunization and it may be treated live bacteria or viruses or dead organisms or their products.

immunoglobulins a group of high molecular weight proteins that act as ANTIBODIES and are present in the SERUM and secretions. Designated Ig, there are five groups each with different functions identified by a particular letter.

Immunoglobulin A (Ig A) is most common and occurs in all secretions of the body. It is the main antibody in the MUCOUS MEMBRANE of the intestines, bronchi, saliva and tears. It defends the body against microorganisms by combining with a protein in the mucosa.

Ig D is found in the serum in small amounts but increases during allergic reactions.

Ig E is found primarily in the lungs, skin and mucous membrane cells and is an anaphylactic antibody (*see* ANAPHYLAXIS).

Ig G is synthesized to combat bacteria and viruses in the body.

Ig M (or macroglobulin) has a very high molecular weight (about five or six times that of the others) and is the first produced by the body when antigens occur. It is also the main antibody in blood group incompatibilities.

immunology the study of immunity, the immune system of the body and all aspects of the body's defence mechanisms.

immunosuppression the use of drugs (immunosuppressives) that affect the body's immune system and lower its resistance to disease. These drugs are used in transplant surgery to maintain the survival of the transplanted organ, and to treat autoimmune diseases. The condition may also be produced as a side effect, e.g. after chemotherapy treatment for cancer. In all instances, there is an increased risk of infection.

immunotherapy the largely experimental technique of developing the body's IMMUNITY to a disease by administering drugs or gradually increasing doses of the appropriate allergens thereby modifying the immune response. The most widely studied disease is cancer where this forms an auxiliary treatment to drug therapy.

impaction a descriptive term for things being locked or wedged together; or stuck in position. For example a wisdom tooth is impacted when it cannot erupt normally because of other tissues blocking it. Also impacted faeces form a block in the colon or rectum and an impacted fracture is where the adjacent ends are locked together.

impetigo a staphylococcal and infectious skin disease found primarily in children. It spreads quickly over the body, starting as a red patch which forms pustules that join to create crusted yellowish sores. It is easily spread by contact or through towels etc. and must be treated quickly otherwise it may continue on an individual for months. Treatment with antibiotics is usually effective.

implant a drug, tissue or artificial object inserted or grafted into the skin or an organ. Drugs are often inserted into the skin for controlled release and in radiotherapy, treatment of prostate tumours, or head/neck cancers can include embedding a capsule of radioactive material in the tissue. A surgical implant covers a tissue graft (e.g. a blood vessel), insertion of a pacemaker or a hip prosthesis.

implantation 1. the placing of an IMPLANT. 2. the attachment of the BLASTOCYST to the uterus wall during the very early stages of embryo development.

impotence when a man is unable to have sexual intercourse through lack of penile ERECTION, or less commonly to ejaculate having gained an erection. The cause may be *organic* and due to a condition or disease (DIABETES, endocrine gland disorder) or more commonly *psychogenic*, i.e. due to psychological or emotional problems such as anxiety, fear, guilt.

incision a surgical cut into tissue or organ, and the act of making the cut.

incisor the tooth with a chisel edge to it, used for biting. They form the four front teeth in each jaw.

incontinence an inability to control bowel movements or passage of urine. Urinary incontinence may be due to a LESION in the brain or spinal cord, injury to the sphincter, or damage to the nerves of the bladder. Stress incontinence occurs during coughing or straining and is common in women due to weakening of muscles through childbirth. There are other categories of incontinence depending on the cause or the frequency of urine passage and the stimulus causing urination.

incubation 1. the time between a person being exposed to an infection and the appearance of symptoms. Incubation periods for diseases tend to be quite constant, some commoner ones being; measles, 10 to 15 days; German measles, 14 to 21; chicken pox, 14 to 21; mumps, 18 to 21 and whooping cough, 7 to 10 days. 2. the time taken to start and grow microorganisms in culture media. 3. the process of caring for a premature baby in an incubator.

incubator 1. the transparent box-like container in which premature babies are kept in controlled, infection-free conditions. 2. a heated container for growth of bacterial cultures in laboratories.

indigestion *see* DYSPEPSIA.

induction the commencement of labour by artificial means, either by administering drugs to produce uterine contractions, or by AMNIOTOMY.

In anaesthesia, it is the process prior to the required state of anaesthesia and includes premedication with a sedative.

infant a child from birth to 12 months.

infarction the formation of an *infarct* or dead area of tissue in an organ or vessel due to the obstruction of the artery supplying blood. The obstruction may be caused by a blood clot or an EMBOLUS.

infection when PATHOGENS invade the body causing disease. Bacteria, viruses, fungi etc. are all included and they enter the body, multiply and after the INCUBATION period symptoms appear. The organisms reach the body in many ways: airborne droplets, direct contact, sexual intercourse, by VECTORS, from contaminated food or drink etc.

infertility when a couple are unable to produce offspring naturally. Female infertility may be because of irregular or no ovulation, blocked FALLOPIAN TUBES, ENDOMETRIOSIS; while a low sperm count or other deficiency in the spermatozoa can lead to male infertility. Treatment can include drug therapy, surgery, or more recently the technique of *in vitro* fertilization.

infestation when animal parasites occur on the skin, in the hair or within the body (e.g. parasitic worms).

inflammation the response of the body's tissues to injury which involves pain, redness, heat and swelling (*acute* inflammation). The first sign when the tissues are infected or injured physically or chemically is a dilation of blood vessels in the affected area increasing blood flow resulting in heat and redness. The circulation then slows a little and white blood cells migrate into the tissues producing the swelling. The white blood cells engulf invading bacteria, dead tissue, foreign particles. After this either the white blood cells migrate back to the circulation, or there is the production and discharge of pus, as healing commences. *Chronic* inflammation is when repair is not complete and there is formation of scar tissue.

influenza a highly infectious disease caused by virus that affects the respiratory tract. Symptoms include headache, weakness and fever, appetite loss and general aches and pains. Sometimes there is the complication of a lung infection which requires immediate treatment. There are three main strains of influenza virus, designated A, B and C. The viruses quickly produce new strains which is why an attack of one is unlikely to provide protection against a later bout of the disease. Epidemics occur periodically and in Britain virus A is responsible for the majority of outbreaks.

ingestion the process of chewing and swallowing food and fluid which then goes into the stomach. Also the means whereby a *phagocyte* (a cell that can surround and break down cell debris, foreign particles and microorganisms) takes in particles.

inhalants substances taken into the body by INHALATION. The substances can be in several forms: inhaling the steam of a hot solution; as a pressurized aerosol of droplets of particles; or as a non-pressurized passive inhaler where powdered medication is drawn into the body by inhaling deeply. Sufferers of asthma use inhalers to deliver drugs to the bronchi (bronchodilator drugs) for relief from attacks.

inhalation 1. (*or* **inspiration**) the act of drawing air into the lungs. 2. the medication breathed in, whether in gas, vapour of particulate form, to ensure contact with and/or treatment of conditions of the throat, bronchi or lungs.

injection the means whereby a liquid (often a drug) is introduced into the body using a syringe when it would otherwise be destroyed by digestive processes. The location of the injection depends upon the speed with which the drug is to be absorbed and the target site. Thus injections may go into the skin (*intradermal*), beneath the skin (*subcutaneous*, as with INSULIN). For slow absorption an *intramuscular* injection would be used, and *intravenous* for fast delivery.

inner ear *see* EAR.

innervation the nerves serving a particular organ, tissue or area of the body which carries MOTOR impulses to the target and sensory impulses away from it and towards the brain.

inoculation the process whereby a small quantity of material is introduced into the body to produce or increase immunity to the disease re-lated to the injected material (*see* IMMUNIZATION *and* VACCINATION).

insemination injection of semen into the vagina whether by sexual intercourse or artificial means (*see* ARTIFICIAL INSEMINATION).

insomnia being unable to remain asleep or to fall asleep in the first instance, resulting in debilitating tiredness. It may be caused by a painful condition but is more likely to be due to anxiety.

insulin a pancreatic hormone produced in the ISLETS OF LANGERHANS that initiates uptake of glucose by body cells and thereby controls the level of glucose in the blood. It works by stimulating proteins on cell surfaces within muscles and other tissues to take up the glucose for their activity. A lack of hormone results in the sugar derived from food being excreted in the urine - the condition DIABETES MELLITUS. For such cases, insulin can be administered by injection.

intercostal the term given to nerves, muscles etc. that are situated between the ribs.

interferon glycoproteins released from cells infected with a virus which restrict, or *interfere* with, the growth of viruses, and they limit the growth of cells, hence their use in cancer treatment (which is as yet of indeterminate value). There are three human interferons: a from white blood cells, b from connective tissue and g from lymphocytes (*see* INTERLEUKINS). Sufficient quantities of interferon can now be produced by GENETIC ENGINEERING.

interleukins one of several cytokines (molecules secreted by a cell to regulate other cells nearby e.g. see IN-

TERFERON) that act between LEUCO-CYTES. There are eight interleukins currently recognized and some are involved in functions such as the recognition of ANTIGENS, enhancing the action of MACROPHAGES and the production of other cytokines e.g. interleukin 2 promotes the production of γ-interferon and is used in the treatment of MELANOMA.

intervertebral disc fibrous cartilaginous discs that connect adjacent vertebrae and permit rotational and bending movements. The discs make up approximately 25% of the backbone length and they act as shock absorbers providing cushioning for the brain and spinal cord. With age the discs lose their effectiveness and may be displaced.

intestinal flora the bacteria usually found in the intestine, some of which synthesize vitamin K. An acidic surrounding is produced by the bacteria and this helps lessen infection by pathogens unable to withstand the acidic conditions.

intestine the part of the ALIMENTARY CANAL or tract between stomach and anus where final digestion and absorption of food matter occur in addition to the absorption of water and production of faeces. The intestine is divided into the small intestine comprising DUODENUM, ILEUM and JEJUNUM, and the large intestine made up of the CAECUM, vermiform APPENDIX, COLON and RECTUM. The length of the intestine in man is about 30 feet.

intolerance when a patient is unable to metabolize a drug. There is usually an associated adverse reaction.

intoxication being poisoned by drugs, alcohol or other toxic substances.

intracranial term meaning within the skull and applied to diseases, structures etc.

intracranial pressure the pressure within the cranium, more specifically the pressure as maintained by all tissues: brain, blood, cerebrospinal fluid etc. An increase in the pressure can occur through injury, haemorrhage, tumour and treatment will be necessary.

intramuscular term meaning within a muscle, as with an intramuscular injection.

intrauterine contraceptive device (IUD) a plastic or metal device, often in the shape of a coil about 25mm long, that is placed in the uterus. The device probably prevents conception by interfering with potential implantation of the embryo. There are sometimes side effects e.g. back pain and heavy menstrual bleeding, but it is a reasonably effective method.

intravenous term meaning relating to the inside of a vein hence intravenous injections are made into a vein, and blood transfusions are intravenous.

intubation the insertion of a tube into the body through a natural opening. It is commonly, though not exclusively, used to keep an airway open by insertion into the mouth or nose into the larynx.

intussusception an eventual obstruction of the bowel caused by one part of the bowel slipping inside another part beneath it, much as a telescope closes up. The commonest sufferers are young children and the symptoms include pain, vomiting and the passage of a jelly-like bloodstained mucus. If the condition does not right itself corrective treatment is essential either by a barium enema or surgery.

invasion when bacteria enter the body; but more commonly used to describe the process whereby malignant cancer cells move into nearby normal and deeper tissues and gain access to the blood vessels.

in vitro referring to a biological or biochemical reaction or process that occurs literally 'in glassware' i.e. in test-tube or a similar piece of laboratory apparatus.

in vitro fertilization (IVF) the process of fertilizing an OVUM outside the body. The technique is used when a woman has blocked FALLOPIAN TUBES or when there is some other reason for sperm and ovum not uniting. The woman produces several ova (due to hormone therapy treatment) which are removed by laparoscopy (*see* LAPAROSCOPE) and these are mixed with sperm and incubated in culture medium until the ova are fertilized and at the BLASTOCYST stage these are implanted in the mother's uterus.

in vivo referring to biological processes that occur in a living organism.

involuntary muscle one of two types of muscle not under voluntary or conscious control such as the blood vessels, stomach and intestines. The heart muscle is slightly different (*see* CARDIAC MUSCLE).

involution the process whereby an organ decreases in size e.g. the return of the uterus to its normal size after childbirth. Also applied to degeneration of organs in old age i.e. atrophy.

iridectomy the surgical removal of part of the IRIS, often undertaken to correct the blockage of aqueous humour (*see* EYE) associated with GLAUCOMA. It may also be necessary for removal of a foreign body or as part of CATARACT surgery.

iridotomy an incision into the IRIS.

iris the part of the EYE that controls the amount of light to enter. It is in effect a muscular disc and to reduce the amount of light entering circular muscles contract, and to increase the aperture in dim light, radiating muscles contract. The varying sized hole is the PUPIL. The iris can be seen through the CORNEA which is transparent and, is the coloured part of the eye, this latter feature is due to pigment cells containing melanin (blue is little; brown is more).

irradiation the use in treatment of any form of radiating energy i.e. electromagnetic radiation in the form of X-rays, α, β or γ radiation, also heat and light. Some radiations are used in diagnosis or cancer treatments, others for relief of pain (heat treatment) etc.

irrigation the washing out of a wound or body cavity with a flow of water or other fluid.

irritable bowel syndrome a condition caused by abnormal muscular contractions (or increased motility) in the COLON producing effects in the large and small intestines. Symptoms include pain in the abdomen which changes location, disturbed bowel movements with diarrhoea then normal movements or constipation, heartburn and a bloated feeling due to wind. The specific cause is unknown and no disease is present.

irritant a general term encompassing any agent that causes irritation of a tissue e.g. nettle stings, chemicals and gases etc.

ischium one of the three bones that comprise each half of the PELVIS. It is the most posterior and it supports the weight of the body when sitting.

islets of Langerhans clusters of cells within the PANCREAS which are the ENDOCRINE part of the gland. There are three types of cells termed alpha, beta and delta, the first two producing GLUCAGON and INSULIN respectively, both vital hormones in the regulation of blood sugar levels. The third hormone produced is somatostatin (also released by the HYPOTHALAMUS) which works antagonistically against growth hormone by blocking its release by the pituitary gland. The islets were named after Paul Langerhans, a German pathologist.

isolation the process whereby a patient with an infectious disease is kept apart from non-infected people. This often includes people who may have contracted the disease but who have yet to show any symptoms. Isolation may also be necessary to ensure a patient does not come into contact with irritating environmental factors.

In *surgery* when a structure or organ is kept apart from all around it through the use of instruments.

J

jaundice a condition characterized by the unusual presence of bile pigment (BILIRUBIN) in the blood. The BILE produced in the liver passes into the blood instead of the intestines and because of this there is a yellowing of the skin and the whites of the eyes.

There are several types of jaundice: *obstructive* due to bile not reaching the intestine due to an obstruction e.g. a GALLSTONE; *haemolytic* where red blood cells are destroyed by HAEMOLYSIS; *hepatocellular* due to a liver disease such as HEPATITIS which results in the liver being unable to use the bilirubin. *Neonatal jaundice* is quite common in newborn infants when the liver is physiologically immature but it usually lasts only a few days. The infant can be exposed to blue light which converts bilirubin to biliverdin, another (harmless) bile pigment.

jejunum the part of the small intestine lying before the ILEUM and after the DUODENUM. Its main function is the absorption of digested food and its lining has numerous finger-like projections (villi) that increase the surface area for absorption. The villi are longer in the jejunum than elsewhere in the small intestine.

joints connections between bones (and cartilages). Joints can be divided upon their structure and the degree to which they permit movement. *Fibrous* joints are fixed by fibrous tissue binding bones together e.g. the bones of the skull. *Cartilaginous* joints are slightly movable. These have discs of cartilage between bones so that only limited movement is permitted over one joint but over several adjacent joints, considerable flexure is achieved, as with the spine. The final category is *synovial* joints which can move freely. Each synovial joint comprises the bones, cartilage over the ends, then a *capsule* (sheath of fibrous tissue) from which the ligaments form, and a SYNOVIAL MEMBRANE with synovial fluid to lubricate the joint.

This type of joint then occurs in two forms: hinge joints allowing planar movement (e.g. the knee) and ball and socket joints permitting all-round movement (e.g. the hip). Joints are subject to various conditions and diseases including SYNOVITIS, epiphysitis (inflammation of the EPIPHYSIS), GOUT, RHEUMATISM and dislocations.

jugular a general term for structures in the neck.

jugular vein any of the veins in the neck, particularly the anterior, internal and external. The anterior jugular vein is an offshoot of the external jugular and runs down the front of the neck. The external jugular itself drains the scalp, face and neck while the larger internal jugular drains the face, neck and brain and is sited vertically down the side of the neck.

K

kaolin (or china clay) a white powder form of aluminium silicate used in cases of skin irritation and as adsorbent taken internally to treat DIARRHOEA.

Kaposi's sarcoma a condition involving malignant skin tumours which form from the blood vessels. Purple lumps, due to the tumours, form on the feet and ankles, spreading to arms and hands. The disease is common in Africa but less so in western countries, although it is associated with AIDS. Radiotherapy is the primary treatment but chemotherapy may also be required.

keloid (*also* **cheloid**) scar tissue which forms due to the growth of fibrous tissue over a burn or injury creating a hard, often raised patch with ragged edges.

keratin a fibrous, sulphur-rich protein made up of coiled polyPEPTIDE chains. It occurs in hair, fingernails and the surface layer of the skin.

keratosis a condition of the skin whereby there is a thickening and overgrowth of the horny layer (or *stratum corneum*) of the SKIN. The condition is usually induced by excessive sunlight and can occur as scales and patchy skin pigmentation (*actinic keratosin*) or as yellow/brown warts (*seborrhoeic keratosis*). It is essential to avoid overexposing skin to sunlight if the condition is to be prevented or treated.

Kernig's sign the inability of someone with MENINGITIS to straighten his legs at the knee when the thighs are at right angles to be body. It is symptomatic of the disease.

ketogenesis the normal production of KETONES in the body due to metabolism of fats. Excess production leads to KETOSIS.

ketone an organic compound that contains a carbonyl group (C=O) within the compound. Ketones can be detected in the body when fat is metabolized for energy when food intake is insufficient.

ketone body one of several compounds (e.g. acetoacetic acid) produced by the liver due to metabolism of fat deposits. These compounds normally provide energy, via KETOGENESIS, for the body's peripheral tissues. In abnormal conditions, when carbohydrate supply is reduced, ketogenesis produces excess ketone bodies in the blood (KETOSIS) which may then appear in the urine (KETONURIA).

ketonuria (acetonuria, or ketoaciduria) the presence of ketone bodies (*see* KETONE and KETONE BODY) in the urine due to starvation or DIABETES MELLITUS causing excessive KETOGENESIS and KETOSIS.

ketosis the build-up of ketones in the body and bloodstream due to a lack of carbohydrates for metabolism, or failure to use fully available carbohydrates resulting in fat breakdown (*see* KETOGENESIS and KETONURIA). It is in-

duced by starvation, DIABETES MELLITUS or any condition in which fats are metabolized quickly and excessively.

kidney one of two glands/organs that remove nitrogenous wastes, mainly UREA, from the blood and also adjust the concentrations of various salts. The kidney measures approximately 10cm long, 6cm wide and 4cm thick, and is positioned at the back of the abdomen, below the diaphragm. Blood is supplied to the kidney by the renal artery and leaves via the renal vein. Each kidney is held in place by fat and connective tissue and comprises an inner medulla and outer cortex. The kidneys produce and eliminate URINE by a complex process of filtration and reabsorption. The 'active' parts are the nephrons which filter blood under pressure, reabsorbing water and other substances. A nephron comprises a renal tubule and blood vessels. The tubule expands into a cup shape (*Bowman's capsule*) that contains a knot of capillaries (the *glomerulus*) and the latter bring the water, urea, salts, etc. Filtrate passes from the glomerulus through three areas of the tubule (proximal convoluted tubule; the loop of Henle, distal convoluted tube, which together form a shape resembling a hairpin) leaving as urine.

kinin one of a group of polyPEPTIDES that lower blood pressure through dilation of the blood vessels and cause SMOOTH MUSCLE to contract. They are associated with inflammation, causing local increases in the permeability of tissue capillaries. In addition they play some part in the allergic response and ANAPHYLAXIS. Kinins do not normally occur in the blood but form under these conditions or when the tissue is damaged (*see also* BRADYKININS).

Klinefelter's syndrome a genetic imbalance in males in which there are 47 rather than 46 CHROMOSOMES, the extra one being an X chromosome producing a genetic make-up of XXY instead of the usual XY. The physical manifestations are small testes which atrophy resulting in a lack of sperm production, enlargement of the breasts, long thin legs and little or no facial or body hair. There may be associated mental retardation and pulmonary disease.

knee the joint connecting the thigh to the lower leg and formed by the femur, tibia and kneecap (PATELLA). It is a hinge type of synovial JOINT with very strong ligaments binding the bones together. Although the knee is a strong joint, it is complex and injuries can be serious.

knee jerk *see* REFLEX ACTION.

knock-knee (*or* **genu valgum**) an abnormal curvature of the legs such that when the knees are touching, the ankles are spaced apart. When walking, the knees knock and severe cases can lead to stress on the joints in the legs, with arthritis. Surgery may be performed to correct the condition which in the past was commonly due to RICKETS but is now due mainly to poor muscles.

Korsakoff's syndrome a neurological disorder described by the Russian neuropsychiatrist Sergei Korsakoff (1854-1900) characterized by short-term memory loss, disorientation and confabulation (the invention and detailed description of events, situations and experiences to cover gaps in the memory). The condition is caused primarily by alcoholism and a deficiency of thiamine (vital in converting carbohydrate to glucose).

kyphosis an abnormal outward curvature of the spine causing the back to be hunched. There is an increased curvature of the spine which may be caused by weak musculature or bad posture (mobile kyphosis) or it may be due to collapsed vertebrae (fixed kyphosis) as in OSTEOPOROSIS of the aged.

L

labia (*singular* **labium**) meaning lips as in the folds of skin enclosing the VULVA (the *labia majora* and *minora*).

labial pertaining to the lips. Also the tooth surface next to the lips.

labour the process of giving birth from dilatation of the CERVIX to expulsion of the afterbirth. It usually commences naturally although some labours are induced (*see* INDUCTION). The cervix expands and at the same time the muscles of the uterus wall contract pushing part of the AMNION down into the opening. The amnion ruptures releasing the 'waters' but these two events do not necessarily occur at the same time. The second stage is the actual delivery of the child which passes through the bony girdle of the pelvis, via the VAGINA to the outside. Initially the head appears at the cervix and the uterine contractions strengthen. These contractions are augmented by abdominal muscular contractions when the baby is in the vagina. When the baby's head is clear, the whole body is helped out and the umbilical cord severed. The final stage, accomplished by some contractions is expulsion of the PLACENTA and membranes.

On average, labour lasts 12 hours (less for subsequent pregnancies) and in the second stage an EPISIOTOMY may be necessary to facilitate the emergence of the head. In most cases, the baby lies head down at delivery although some are delivered feet or buttocks first (BREECH PRESENTATION). Other complications tend to be rare and maternal mortality is very low in the west.

labyrinth part of the inner ear (*see* EAR) consisting of canals, ducts and cavities forming the organs of hearing and balance. There are two parts; the *membranous labyrinth* comprising the semicircular canals and associated structures and the central cavity of the cochlea, and the *bony labyrinth*, a system of canals filled with perilymph and surrounding the other parts.

laceration a wound with jagged edges.

lacrimal relating to, or about tears.

lacrimal gland one of a pair of glands situated above and to the side of each eye that secrete saline and slightly alkaline tears that moisten the conjunctiva (the mucous membrane lining the inside of the eyelid). The glands comprise part of the *lacrimal apparatus*, the remainder being the lacrimal ducts (or canaliculi) through which the tears drain, to the lacrimal sacs and the nasal cavity.

lactation the process of milk secretion by the MAMMARY GLANDS in the breast which begins at the end of pregnancy. COLOSTRUM is produced and secreted before the milk. Lactation is controlled by hormones and stops when the baby ceases to be breast fed.

lactase the enzyme that acts on milk sugar (LACTOSE) to produce glucose and galactose.

lacteal vessels forming part of the lymphatic system. They occur as projections with a closed end extending into villi (*see* VILLUS) in the small intestine and take up digested fats as a milky fluid called chyle.

lactose milk sugar found only in mammalian milk and produced by the MAMMARY GLANDS. It is made up of one molecule of glucose and one molecule of galactose. People with a low level of activity of the enzyme LACTASE, or none at all, cannot absorb lactose, a condition called lactose intolerance.

lacuna (*plural* **lacunae**) an anatomical term meaning a small depression, cavity or pit, especially in compact bone.

laminectomy the surgical procedure

in which access is gained to the spinal cord by the removal of the arch of one or more vertebrae. It is adopted when a tumour is to be removed, or a slipped disc is to be treated.

lancet a surgical knife that is small and pointed and sharp on both edges.

lanugo a fine, downy hair that covers the foetus between the fifth and ninth months. It is lost in the ninth month and is thus seen only on babies born prematurely.

laparoscope a type of ENDOSCOPE with a light source and a means of viewing the object, that is inserted into the abdominal cavity through a small incision. This allows a surgeon to view the organs in the cavity and a laparoscope is also used to enable some minor operations to be performed using instruments inserted through a second incision.

laparoscopy the use of a LAPAROSCOPE to examine the organs in the abdominal cavity. Carbon dioxide is injected into the cavity to expand it before the laparoscope is inserted. In addition to being used purely for observation, a laparoscopy is also useful for taking a biopsy, sterilizations, and for collecting ova for IN VITRO FERTILIZATION.

laparotomy a general term for any incision into the abdominal cavity. Types of laparotomy include COLOSTOMY, APPENDICECTOMY etc.

large intestine *see* INTESTINE.

laryngectomy surgical excision of all or part of the LARYNX. This procedure is adopted for cancer of the larynx.

laryngitis inflammation of the mucous membrane that lines the LARYNX and vocal cords. It is due to viral infection in the main, but also bacteria,

chemical irritants, heavy smoking or excessive use of the voice. *Acute* laryngitis accompanies infections of the upper respiratory tract and the symptoms include pain, a cough, difficulty in swallowing. *Chronic* laryngitis may be due to recurrence of the acute form, but is often attributable to excessive smoking worsened by alcohol. Changes occurring in the vocal cords are more permanent and the symptoms are as for the acute form, but longer lasting.

laryngoscope a type of endoscope used to examine the larynx.

laryngotracheobronchitis an acute inflammation of the major parts of the respiratory tract, causing shortness of breath, a croup-like cough and hoarseness. It occurs usually through viral infection and particularly in young children where there may be some obstruction of the LARYNX (*see also* CROUP). The main airways, bronchi, become coated with fluid generated by the inflamed tissues resulting in the shortness of breath. Treatment is through inhalations, antibiotics if appropriate and if the obstruction is serious, hospitalization may be necessary for INTUBATION, TRACHEOSTOMY etc.

larynx part of the air passage connecting the PHARYNX with the TRACHEA and also the organ producing vocal sounds. It is situated high up in the front of the neck and is constructed of cartilages with ligaments and muscles. The ligaments bind together the cartilages and one pair of these form the VOCAL CORDS. The larynx is lined with mucous membrane and in all is about 5cm long.

laxative a substance that is taken to

evacuate the bowel or to soften stools. Typical laxatives include castor oil, senna, and its derivatives (*see also* PURGATIVE).

Legionnaire's disease a bacterial infection and a form of pneumonia caused by *Legionella pneumophila*. It produces an illness similar to influenza with symptoms appearing after a two to ten day incubation period. Fever, chills, head and muscular aches may progress to PLEURISY and chest pains. Antibiotic treatment is usually effective (e.g. erythromycin).

The disease was named after an outbreak in America in 1976 at the American Legion convention. The bacterium is found in nature, particularly in water, and static water provides ideal conditions for multiplication. Inhalation of an aerosol of water is the likeliest way of becoming infected and air conditioning cooling towers are a particular source of infected water. It is vital that infected systems be cleaned and chlorinated.

lens the part of the eye that focuses incoming light onto the RETINA. It is composed of a fibrous protein, crystallin, and is enclosed in a thin capsule.

leprosy a serious disease caused by the bacterium *Mycobacterium leprae* that attacks the skin, nerves and mucous membranes and has an incubation period of several years. There are two forms of the disease, *tuberculoid* and *lepromatous*, depending upon the resistance of the host (the former occurs in those with a higher degree of immunity). The tuberculoid form produces discoloured patches of skin with some numbness

but is generally benign and often heals untreated.

Lepromatous leprosy is a much more serious and progressively destructive form of the disease, creating lumps in the skin, thickening of skin and nerves, inflammation of the iris, numbness of the skin with muscle weakness and paralysis. The more serious cases show deformity and considerable disfigurement and sometimes blindness. There is also an intermediate form with symptoms of both types (indeterminate leprosy).

Although many millions of people are affected, drugs therapy is quite effective, providing a combination of antibiotics is used (because the bacterium develops resistance to one of the sulphone drugs commonly used).

leptomeningitis inflammation of two of the three MENINGES surrounding the brain and spinal cord. Specifically, the inner two (pia mater and arachnoid) are affected.

leptospirosis an acute infectious disease caused by bacteria in the genus *Leptospira*. The disease varies from the mild form of an influenza type of illness to the more serious cases involving fever, liver disease and therefore jaundice, and possibly kidney disease or meningitis. In such cases there may be fatalities. The organism occurs in the urine of rats and dogs and this renders workers on farms, sewage works etc. more susceptible, but it can be contracted by bathing or immersion in contaminated water (e.g. canals). Antibiotics can be given but must be administered at an early stage to be effective.

One particular species *L. icterohaemorrhagiae*, which is transmitted by rats, is responsible for the type called Weil's disease.

lesion a wound or injury to body tissues. Also an area of tissue which because of damage due to disease or wounding does not function fully. Thus primary lesions include tumours and ulcers, and from primary lesions secondaries may form.

leucocyte (or leukocyte) a white blood cell, so called because it contains no HAEMOGLOBIN. It also differs from red blood cells in having a nucleus. Leucocytes are formed in the bone marrow, spleen, thymus and lymph nodes and there are three types: granulocytes, comprising 70% of all white blood cells, lymphocytes (25%) and monocytes (5%). Granulocytes help combat bacterial and viral infection and may be involved in allergies. LYMPHOCYTES destroy foreign bodies either directly or through production of antibodies and MONOCYTES ingest bacteria and foreign bodies by the process called *phagocytosis* (engulfing microorganisms and cell debris to remove them from the body). In disease, immature forms of leucocytes may appear in the blood (ultimately forming both red and white blood cells).

leucocytosis except for pregnancy, menstruation and during exercise an abnormal and temporary increase in the number of white blood cells in the blood. It usually accompanies bacterial but not viral infections, because the body's defence mechanism is fighting the bacteria by producing leucocytes. A blood sample may thus form a useful diagnostic tool for a condition which has not yet manifested any physical symptoms.

leucorrhea a discharge of white or yellow-coloured mucus from the vagina. It may be a normal condition, increasing before and after menstruation but a large discharge probably indicates an infection somewhere in the genital tract. A common cause is the infection called THRUSH but it may also be due to GONORRHOEA in which case the treatment will differ.

leukaemia a cancerous disease in which there is an uncontrolled proliferation of LEUCOCYTES in the bone marrow. The cells fail to mature to adult cells and thus cannot function as part of the defence mechanism against infections. This leads to anaemia, bleeding, easy bruising, with enlargement of the spleen, liver and lymph nodes. Acute leukaemia has a sudden onset and development while the chronic form may take years to develop the same symptoms.

The cause of leukaemia is unknown although it has been attributed to viruses, exposure to toxic chemicals or ionizing radiations. In addition to the acute and chronic forms, it is further classified by the predominant white blood cells thus acute lymphoblastic leukaemia, acute myeloblastic leukaemia (myeloblast is an early form of granulocytes, *see* LEUCOCYTE), chronic lymphatic leukaemia. The treatment involves radiotherapy, chemotherapy and bone marrow transplants and although there is no cure, the outlook has improved over recent years. The survival or remission rate varies with the type of leukaemia.

libido the sexual drive, often associated with psychiatric illnesses. Lack of libido may be due to illness or a lack of sex hormones due to an endocrine disorder.

Librium a minor tranquillizer used in the treatment of anxiety. It is taken orally and relaxes muscles although there are side effects such as nausea and skin reactions.

lice (*singular* **louse**) insects parasitic on man. Lice are wingless and attach themselves to hair or clothing by means of their legs and claws. They suck blood and are particularly resistant to crushing and have to be removed using special shampoos and combs (*see also* PEDICULOSIS).

ligament bands of fibrous connective tissue composed chiefly of COLLAGEN, that join bones together, restricting movement and preventing dislocation. Ligaments strengthen joints and most joints are surrounded by a capsular ligament. Also, a layer of SEROUS MEMBRANE e.g. the PERITONEUM that supports or links organs.

ligation the procedure of tying off a duct or blood vessel to prevent flow during surgery etc. The application of a LIGATURE.

ligature material for tying firmly around a blood vessel or duct to stop bleeding or prevent flow. The material may be wire, silk, catgut etc.

lightening a sensation experienced by many pregnant women, normally towards the last month of the pregnancy, whereby the foetus settles lower in the pelvis. This lessens the pressure on the diaphragm and breathing becomes easier.

light reflex the mechanism whereby the PUPIL of the EYE opens in response to direct light or consensual pupillary stimulation (i.e. stimulation of one pupil with light results in a response from the other pupil).

lignocaine a commonly used local anaesthetic. It is given by injection for minor surgery and dental treatment and it can be applied directly to the eyes, throat etc. because it is absorbed directly through mucous membranes. It is also used in the treatment of some disorders in heart rhythm.

linctus a medicine, particularly to treat coughs, that is thick and syrup-like.

lingual term meaning relating to the tongue, or something close to the tongue e.g. lingual nerve, or the lingual surface of a tooth.

liniment a creamy/oily substance for rubbing onto the skin to alleviate irritation or pain. Many of the compounds are poisonous and contain such substances as camphor, turpentine and even belladonna.

linkage two or more GENES are said to be linked together if they occur close to each other on the same CHROMOSOME. The genes are thus likely to be inherited together as will be characteristics that they represent. This is because the linked genes are more likely to be together in nuclei formed as a result of meiosis (the chromosomal division that produces the GAMETES).

lipolysis the breakdown of lipids into FATTY ACIDS via the action of the enzyme lipase.

lipoma a benign tumour made up of fat cells which can occur in the fibrous tissues of the body, often beneath the skin. The only problem associated with such structures may be their size and position.

liposarcoma a malignant tumour of fat cells which is very rare, particularly under the age of 30. It occurs in the buttocks or thighs.

liposome a spherical droplet of microscopic size comprising fatty membranes around an aqueous vesicle. Liposomes are created in the laboratory by adding an aqueous solution to a phospholipid gel (phospholipids are compounds containing FATTY ACIDS and a phosphate group). Liposomes bear some resemblance to living cell components and are studied on this basis. Additionally, they can be introduced into living cells and are used to transport toxic drugs to a specific treatment site. The liposomes retain the drug while in the blood and on passing through the chosen organ the membrane is melted by selectively heating the organ and the drug is released. This technique is used for certain forms of cancer.

listeriosis an infectious disease caused when the Gram-positive (*see* GRAM'S STAIN) bacterium *Listeria monocytogenes* which attacks animals is contracted by man through eating infected products. It produces symptoms similar to influenza or it may cause MENINGITIS or ENCEPHALITIS. The old and frail are more susceptible as are the newborn. It may terminate a pregnancy or damage the foetus if contracted during a pregnancy. Antibiotics such as penicillin provide an effective treatment.

Little's disease CEREBRAL PALSY on both sides of the body but where the legs are affected more than the arms.

liver a very important organ of the body, with many functions critical in regulating metabolic processes. It is also the largest gland in the body weighing around 1kg. It occupies the top right hand part of the abdominal cavity and is made up of four lobes. It is fastened to the abdominal wall by ligaments and sits beneath the DIAPHRAGM, and upon the right kidney, large intestine, DUODENUM and stomach.

There are two blood vessels supplying the liver: the hepatic artery delivers oxygenated blood, while the hepatic portal vein conveys digested food from the stomach. Among its functions, the liver converts excess glucose to GLYCOGEN for storage as a food reserve; excess amounts of AMINO ACIDS are converted to urea for excretion by the kidneys; BILE is produced for storage in the GALL BLADDER and LIPOLYSIS occurs; some poisons are broken down (detoxified) hence the beneficial effect of the hepatic portal vein carrying blood to the liver rather than it going around the body first.

The liver also synthesizes blood-clotting substances such as FIBRINOGEN and prothrombin and the anticoagulant HEPARIN; it breaks down red blood cells at the end of their life and processes the haemoglobin for iron, which is stored; vitamin A is synthesized and stored and it also stores vitamins B_{12}, D, E and K. In the embryo it forms red blood cells. Such is the chemical and biochemical activity of the liver that significant heat energy is generated and this organ is a major contributor of heat to the body.

lobe certain organs are divided by fissures into large divisions which are called lobes, e.g. the brain, liver and lungs.

lobectomy the removal of a lobe of an organ e.g. lung or brain. A lobe of a lung may be removed for cancer or other disease.

lobotomy in general, cutting a lobe. More specifically, a neurosurgical operation rarely performed now which involved severing the nerve fibres in the frontal lobe of the brain. It was performed to reduce severe depression or emotional conditions but produced serious side effects such as epilepsy and personality changes. Modern techniques permit the production of small LESIONS in specific areas and side effects are rare.

lobule a small lobe. Also a division of an organ that is smaller than a lobe, e.g. the lobules of the liver.

lochia the material discharged through the vagina from the uterus after childbirth and which takes a few weeks. Initially it consists mainly of blood, then it becomes more mucus but with some blood and then a whitish mixture of cell fragments and microbes.

lockjaw see TETANUS.

locomotor ataxia an unsteady gait which is one symptom of TABES DORSALIS, a form of SYPHILIS. The organism destroys sensory nerves producing further symptoms such as pains in the legs and body, loss of bladder control and blurred vision due to optic nerve damage.

loin that area of the back between the lower ribs and pelvis.

lumbago pain of any sort in the lower back. It can be muscular, skeletal or neurological in origin. A severe case may be due to a strained muscle or

slipped disc and the latter is usually the cause of lumbago with SCIATICA.

lumbar a general term for anything relating to the LOINS, e.g. lumbar vertebra.

lumbar puncture the procedure whereby a hollow needle is inserted into the spinal canal in the lumbar region (usually between the third and fourth lumbar vertebrae) to obtain a sample of cerebrospinal fluid. The fluid is used in diagnosis of diseases of the nervous system, or to introduce drugs, anaesthetics, etc.

lumbar vertebrae numbering five, the lumbar vertebrae are between the SACRUM and the thoracic vertebrae at the lowest part of the back. These vertebrae are not fused and have strong attachments points (processes) for the muscles of the lower back.

lumpectomy the surgical removal of a tumour with the tissue immediately around it but leaving intact the bulk of the tissue and the lymph nodes. This applies particularly to breast cancer when the procedure is often followed by radiotherapy and is undertaken for patients with a small tumour (less than 2cm) and no metastases (see METASTASIS) to nearby lymph nodes or organs elsewhere in the body.

lungs the sac-like, paired organs of respiration situated with their base on the DIAPHRAGM and the top projecting into the neck. Each lung consists of fibrous, elastic sacs that are convoluted to provide a large surface area for gaseous exchange. Air enters the body through the windpipe or TRACHEA which branches into two bronchi (see BRONCHUS), one to each lung. Further branching then occurs, into numerous BRONCHIOLES. The bronchioles divide further and then end in alveoli (*see* ALVEOLUS) which are tiny sac-like structures where the gaseous exchange occurs. The exchange of oxygen and carbon dioxide occurs between the many blood capillaries on one side of the membrane and the air on the other. The lungs are served by the pulmonary arteries and pulmonary veins.

The *total lung capacity* of an adult male is five to six litres although only about half a litre (500ml) is exchanged in normal breathing (called the *tidal volume*).

Lyme disease an arthritic disease with rashes, fever and possibly carditis (inflammation of the heart) and EN-CEPHALITIS. It is caused by a spirochaete (a type of BACTERIUM) that is transmitted by tick bite. Symptoms may not appear until some time after the bite but antibiotics can be used in treatment.

lymph a colourless, watery fluid that surrounds the body tissues and circulates in the lymphatic system. It is derived from blood and is similar to plasma comprising 95% water, with protein, sugar, salts and LYM-PHOCYTES. The lymph is circulated by muscular action and it passes through LYMPH NODES which act as filters, and is eventually returned to the blood via the thoracic duct (one of the two main vessels of the lymphatic system).

lymphadenectomy removal of LYMPH NODES when, for example, a node has become cancerous due to it draining the area around an organ with a malignancy.

lymphadenitis inflammation of the LYMPH NODES which become enlarged, hard and tender. The neck lymph nodes are commonly affected in association with another inflammatory condition.

lymphadenoma *see* HODGKIN'S DIS-EASE.

lymphangiography the technique of injecting a radio-opaque substance into the lymphatic system to render it visible on an X-ray, used primarily in investigating the spread of cancer.

lymphatic gland *see* GLAND.

lymphatics (*or* **lymphatic system**) the network of vessels, valves, nodes etc. that carry lymph from the tissues to the bloodstream and help maintain the internal fluid environment of the body. Lymph drains into capillaries and larger vessels, passing through nodes and going eventually into two large vessels (the thoracic duct and right lymphatic duct) which return it to the bloodstream by means of the innominate veins.

lymph node small oval structures that occur at various points in the LYMPHATICS. They are found grouped in several parts of the body, including the neck, groin and armpit and their main functions are to remove foreign particles and produce LYMPHOCYTES, important in the IM-MUNE response.

lymphocyte a type of white blood cell (LEUCOCYTE) produced in the bone marrow and also present in the SPLEEN, THYMUS GLAND and lymph nodes, which forms a vital component of the immune system. There are two types: B cells and T cells. B cells produce antibodies and search out and bind with particular antigens. T cells circulate through the thymus gland where they differentiate. When they contact an antigen, large numbers of T cells are generated which secrete chemical compounds to assist the B cells in destroying, e.g. bacteria.

lymphocytosis when the blood contains an increased number of lymphocytes as during many diseases or lymphocytic LEUKAEMIA.

lymphoedema the build-up of LYMPH in soft tissues causing swelling. It may be due to obstruction of the vessels by parasites, tumour or inflammation. A secondary form of lymphoedema may occur after removal of lymph vessels in surgery, or by blocking. The condition occurs most in the legs and treatment comprises use of elastic bandages and DIURETIC drugs.

lymphography see LYMPHANGIOGRAPHY.

lymphoid tissue tissues that are involved in the formation of lymph, lymphocytes and antibodies such as the spleen, thymus and lymph nodes.

lymphoma a tumour, usually malignant, of the lymph nodes. Often several lymph nodes become enlarged and subsequent symptoms include fever, anaemia, weakness and weight loss. If much of the lymphoid tissue is involved, there may be enlargement of the liver and spleen. Life expectancy is often very low although treatment with drugs often produces a marked response. Radiotherapy may be used for localized varieties (*see also* HODGKIN'S DISEASE).

lymphosarcoma a tumour of the lymphatics resulting in enlargement of the glands, spleen and liver. In general an older term applied to lymphomas other than HODGKIN'S DISEASE.

lysis the destruction of cells by antibodies called *lysins*, thus haemolysis is the break-up of red blood cells by haemolysin. Also, more generally, the destruction of cells or tissues due to breakdown of the cell membranes.

lysozyme an enzyme present in tears, nasal secretions and on the skin that has an antibacterial action (by breaking the cell wall of the bacterium). Lysozyme also occurs in egg white.

M

macrocephaly an abnormal enlargement of the head when compared with the rest of the body, *see* MICROCEPHALY, HYDROCEPHALUS.

macrocyte a red blood cell (erythrocyte) which is abnormally large. Macrocytes are characteristic of PERNICIOUS ANAEMIA.

macrocytosis the condition in which abnormally large red blood cells (erythrocytes) are present in the blood. It is characteristic of macrocytic anaemias such as those caused by the deficiency of vitamin B_{12} (*see* CYANOCOBALAMIN and PERNICIOUS ANAEMIA) and folic acid.

Macrocytes are also produced in those anaemias in which there is an increased rate of production of erythrocytes.

macrophage a large scavenger cell (PHAGOCYTE), numbers of which are found in various tissues and organs including the LIVER, SPLEEN, BONE MARROW, LYMPH NODES, CONNECTIVE TISSUE and the *microglia* of the CENTRAL NERVOUS SYSTEM. They remove foreign bodies such as bacteria from blood and tissues. *Fixed macrophages* remain in one place in the connective tissue, *free microphages* are able to migrate between cells and gather at sites of infection to remove bacteria and other foreign material.

macula a small area or spot of tissue that is distinct from the surrounding region e.g. the *yellow spot* in the retina of the eye.

macules spots of small pigmented areas in the skin which may be thickened. They appear as a result of pregnancy, sunburn, eczema, psoriasis and may be symptomatic of other diseases such as syphilis and those affecting internal organs.

malabsorption syndrome a group of diseases in which there is a reduction in the normal absorption of digested food materials in the small intestine. The food materials involved are commonly fats, vitamins, minerals, amino acids and iron. The diseases include COELIAC DISEASE, PANCREATITIS, CYSTIC FIBROSIS, SPRUE and STAGNANT LOOP SYNDROME and also surgical removal of a part of the small intestine.

malaria an infectious disease caused by the presence of minute parasitic

organisms of the genus *Plasmodium* in the blood. The disease is characterized by recurrent bouts of fever and anaemia, the interval between the attacks depending upon the species . The parasite is transmitted to man by the *Anopheles* mosquito, (common in sub-tropical and tropical regions) being present in the salivary glands and passed into the bloodstream of a person when the insect bites. Similarly, the parasite is ingested by the mosquito when it takes a blood meal from an infected person. Efforts to control malaria have centred on destruction of the mosquito and its breeding sites. Once injected into the blood, the organisms concentrate in the liver where they multiply and then re-enter the bloodstream destroying red blood cells. This releases the parasites causing shivering, fever, sweating and anaemia. The process is then repeated, with hours or days between attacks. Drugs are used both to prevent infection, although these may not be totally effective, and to cure the disease once present.

malignant a term used in several ways but commonly referring to a tumour that proliferates rapidly and destroys surrounding healthy tissue, and which can spread via the lymphatic and blood system to other parts of the body. The term is also applied to a more serious form of a disease than the usual one which is life-threatening such as *malignant smallpox* and malignant HYPERTENSION.

malnutrition a condition caused either by an unbalanced diet, i.e. too much of one type of food at the expense of others or by an inadequate food intake (*subnutrition*) which can lead to starvation. The condition may also arise due to internal disfunction e.g. MALABSORPTION or other *metabolic* disturbance within the body.

malposition (*and* **malpresentation**) the situation in which the head of an unborn baby before and near delivery is not in the usual (occipitoanterior) position. In *malposition* the baby is head down but a wider part of the skull is presented to the pelvic opening due to the angle of the head. In *malpresentation* the baby is not head down. Both these conditions prolong and complicate labour and, in the latter case especially, are likely to require delivery by CAESARIAN SECTION.

mammary gland a gland present in the female breast which produces milk after childbirth.

mammography a special X-ray technique used to determine the structure of the breast and useful in the early detection of tumours and in distinguishing between benign and malignant tumours.

mammoplasty plastic surgery of the breasts to decrease or increase size and other shape.

mania a mental illness characterized by great excitement and euphoria which then gives way to irritability as in MANIC DEPRESSIVE PSYCHOSIS.

manic depressive psychosis a form of severe mental illness in which there are alternating bouts of MANIA and severe DEPRESSION. While manic the person may be incoherent, outrageous or violent. Drug treatment is required for both phases of the illness, and may reduce the frequency of attacks.

mantoux test a test for the presence of a measure of immunity to tuberculosis. A protein called *tuberculin*, extracted from the tubercle bacilli (bacteria) is injected in a small quantity beneath the skin of the forearm. If an inflamed patch appears within 18 to 24 hours it indicates that a measure of immunity is present and that the person has been exposed to tuberculosis. The size of the reaction indicates the severity of the original tuberculosis infection although it does not mean that the person is actively suffering from the disease at that time.

marasmus a wasting condition in infants usually due to defective feeding. The child has a low body weight (less than 75% of normal), lacks skin fat and is pale and apathetic. Various disorders and diseases can bring this about including prolonged vomiting and diarrhoea, organ disease, e.g. of the heart, kidneys and lungs; infections and parasitic diseases and MALABSORPTION. Treatment depends upon the cause but the provision and gradual increase of nourishment and fluids is always of primary importance.

Marfan's syndrome an inherited disease of the connective tissue producing defects in the skeleton, heart and eyes. The person is abnormally tall and thin; having spindly, elongated fingers and toes (arachnodactyly) spine and chest deformities and weak ligaments. Heart defects include a hole in the septum separating the right and left atrium (*atrial septal defect*) and narrowing of the AORTA (coarction of the aorta). The lenses of the eyes are partially dislocated.

mastalgia pain in the breast.

mast cell a large cell, many of which are found in loose connective tissue. The cytoplasm contains numerous granules with chemicals important in the body including histamine, serotonin, heparin and the antibody immunoglobulin E. All are important in allergic and inflammatory responses.

mastectomy surgical removal of the breast usually performed because of the presence of a tumour. Mastectomy may be *simple* leaving the skin (and possibly the nipple) so that an artificial breast (prosthesis) can be inserted. Or it may be *radical* in which case the whole breast, pectoral muscles and lymph nodes beneath the armpit are all removed, generally performed because a cancer has spread.

mastication chewing of food in the mouth, the first stage in the digestive process.

mastitis inflammation of the breast usually caused by bacterial infection during breast feeding, the organisms responsible gaining access through cracked nipples. *Cystic mastitis* does not involve inflammation, but the presence of cysts (thought to be caused by hormonal factors), causes the breast(s) to be lumpy.

mastoidectomy surgical removal of the inflamed cells in the MASTOID PROCESS of the temporal bone of the skull, which is situated behind the ear, when these have become infected. *See* MASTOIDITIS.

mastoiditis inflammation of the mastoid cells and mastoid antrum usually caused by bacterial infection which spreads from the middle ear. Treatment is by means of antibiotic drugs and sometimes surgery. *See* MASTOID PROCESS and MASTOIDECTOMY.

mastoid process a *breast-like* projection of the temporal bone of the skull which contains numerous air spaces (mastoid cells) and is situated behind the ear. It provides a point of attachment for some of the neck muscles and communicates with the middle ear through an air-filled channel called the *mastoid antrum*. *See* MASTOIDITIS.

measles an extremely infectious disease of children caused by a virus and characterized by the presence of a rash. It occurs in epidemics every two or three years. After an incubation period of 10 to 15 days the initial symptoms are those of a cold with coughing, sneezing and high fever. It is at this stage that the disease is most infectious and spreads from one child to another in airborne droplets before measles has been diagnosed. This is the main factor responsible for the epidemic nature of the disease. Small red spots with a white centre (known as *Koplik spots*) may appear in the mouth on the inside of the cheeks. Then a characteristic rash develops on the skin, spreading from behind the ears and across the face and also affecting other areas. The small red spots may be grouped together in patches and the child's fever is usually at its height while these are developing. The spots and fever gradually decline and no marks are left upon the skin, most children making a good recovery. However, complications can occur, particularly pneumonia and middle ear infections, which can result in deafness. A vaccine now available has reduced the incidence and severity of measles in the United Kingdom.

meatus a passage or opening, e.g. the *external auditory meatus* linking the *pinna* of the outer ear to the eardrum.

meconium the first stools of a new-born baby which are dark green and slimy and contain bile pigments, mucus and debris from cells and passed during the first two days after birth.

media the middle layer of a tissue or organ. Usually it is applied to the middle layer of the wall of a vein or artery comprising alternating sheaths of smooth muscle and elastic fibres.

mediastinum the space in the chest cavity between the two lungs which contains the heart, aorta, oesophagus, trachea, thymus gland and phrenic nerves.

medication any substance introduced into or on the body for the purposes of medical treatment, e.g. drugs and medicated dressings.

medulla refers to the inner portion of a tissue or organ when there are two distinct parts. Examples include the adrenal medulla and the medulla of the kidneys. *Compare* CORTEX.

medulla oblongata the lowest part of the brain stem which extends through the FORAMEN *magnum* to become the upper part of the spinal cord. It contains important centres which govern respiration, circulation, swallowing and salivation.

megaloblast an abnormally large form of any of the cells that go on to produce erythrocytes (red blood cells). In certain forms of anaemia (megaloblastic anaemias) they are found in the bone marrow and their presence is due to a deficiency of vitamin B_{12} or of folic acid. They indicate a failure in the maturation process of erythrocytes which results in anaemia.

meiosis a type of cell division which occurs in the maturation process of the gametes (sperm and ova) so that the sex cells eventually contain only half the number of chromosomes of the parent cells from which they are derived. The daughter cells also have genetic variation from the parent cell, brought about by a process known as 'crossing over' which occurs during meiosis. When sperm and ovum fuse at fertilization, the full chromosome number is restored in a unique combination in the embryo. There are two phases of division in meiosis each of which is divided into four stages namely *prophase, metaphase, anaphase* and *telophase.*

melanin a dark brown pigment found in the skin and hair and also in the choroid layer of the eye. Melanin is contained and produced within cells known as *melanocytes* in the dermis layer of the skin. When the skin is exposed to hot sunshine, more melanin is produced giving a 'suntan.' In dark-skinned races more melanin is produced by greater activity of the melanocytes and it helps to protect the skin from harmful ultra violet radiation.

melanoma an extremely malignant tumour of the melanocytes, the cells in the skin which produce melanin. Melanomas are also found, although less commonly, in the mucous membranes and in the eye. There is a link between the occurrence of melanoma of the skin and exposure to harmful ultra violet light during sunbathing. A highly malignant form can also arise from the pigmented cells of moles. Melanoma can be successfully treated by surgery if it is superficial and caught at an early stage. However, it commonly spreads, especially to the liver and lymph nodes, in which case the outlook is poor. The incidence of malignant melanoma is increasing and has attracted much attention in connection with the formation of holes in the ozone layer, which screens the earth from harmful UV radiation. Most experts recommend that people should cover exposed skin, use sunscreen creams and avoid the sun at the hottest part of the day .

membrane a thin composite layer of lipoprotein surrounding an individual cell or a thin layer of tissue surrounding an organ, lining a cavity or tube or separating tissues and organs within the body.

memory the function of the brain which enables past events to be stored and remembered. It is a highly complex function which probably involves many areas of the brain including the temporal lobes. Memory involves three stages comprising registration, storage and recall (of information). Information is committed either to the short term or long term memory. Most forgetfulness involves the retrieval of information, and memory of a particular item is improved if the context in which it was registered and stored can be recreated. This technique is used by the Police when trying to gain information from witnesses in the field of reconstruction of a crime.

Menière's disease a disease first described by the Frenchman, Prosper Menière in 1861, which affects the inner ear causing deafness and TINNITUS (ringing in the ears), vertigo, vomiting and sweating. The disease is most common in middle-aged men, with severe attacks of vertigo followed by vomiting. The time interval between attacks varies from one week to several months, but the deafness gradually becomes more pronounced. The symptoms are caused by an over-accumulation of fluid in the labyrinths of the inner ears, but the reason for this is not known. Treatment is by a variety of drugs and surgery, neither of which are completely successful.

meninges the three connective tissue membranes which surround the spinal cord and brain. The outermost layer (meninx) is called the *dura mater* which is fibrous, tough and inelastic, and also called the *pachymeninx*, closely lining the inside of the skull and helping to protect the brain. It is thicker than the middle layer, the *arachnoid mater*, which surrounds the brain. The innermost layer, the *pia mater*, is thin and delicate and lines the brain. Cerebrospinal fluid circulates between it and the arachnoid mater and both these inner layers are richly supplied with blood vessels which supply the surface of the brain and skull. These two inner membranes are sometimes collectively called the *pia-arachnoid* or *leptomeninges*.

meningioma a slow-growing tumour affecting the MENINGES of the brain or spinal cord which exerts pressure on the underlying nervous tissue. It may cause paraplegia if present in the spinal cord or other losses of sensation.

In the brain it causes increasing neurological disability. A meningioma can be present for many years without being detected. The usual treatment is surgical removal if the tumour is accessible. Malignant meningiomas, known as *meningeal sarcomas*, can invade surrounding tissues. These are treated by means of surgery and also radiotherapy.

meningitis inflammation of the meninges (membranes) of the brain (*cerebral meningitis*) or spinal cord (*spinal meningitis*) or the disease may affect both regions. Meningitis may affect the *dura mater* membrane in which case it is known as *pachymeningitis*, although this is relatively uncommon. It often results as a secondary infection due to the presence of disease elsewhere, as in the case of *tuberculous meningitis* and *syphilitic meningitis*. Meningitis which affects the other two membranes, (the *pia-arachnoid* membranes) is known as *leptomeningitis* and this is more common and may be either a primary or secondary infection. Meningitis is also classified according to its causal organism and may be either viral or bacterial. *Viral meningitis* is fairly mild and as it does not respond to drugs, treatment is by means of bed rest until recovery takes place. *Bacterial meningitis* is much more common and is caused by the organisms responsible for tuberculosis, pneumonia and syphilis. Also, the *meningococcus* type of bacteria causes one of the commonest forms of the disease, *meningococcal meningitis*. The symptoms are a severe headache, sensitivity to light and sound, muscle rigidity especially affecting the neck, KERNIG'S SIGN, vomiting, paralysis, coma and death. These are caused by inflammation of the meninges and by a rise in INTRACRANIAL PRESSURE. One of the features of meningitis is that there is a change in the constituents and appearance of the cerebrospinal fluid, and the infective organism can usually be isolated from it and identified. The onset of the symptoms can be very rapid and death can also follow swiftly. Treatment is by means of antibiotic drugs and sulphonamides.

menopause also known as the climacteric this is the time in a woman's life when the ovaries no longer release an egg cell every month and ceases. The woman is normally no longer able to bear a child and the age at which the menopause occurs is usually between 45 to 55. The menopause may be marked by a gradual decline in menstruation or in its frequency, or it may cease abruptly. There is a disturbance in the balance of sex hormones and this causes a number of physical symptoms including palpitations, hot flushes, sweats, vaginal dryness, loss of libido and depression. In the long term, there is a gradual loss of bone (OSTEOPOROSIS) in postmenopausal women which leads to greater risk of fractures, especially of the femur in the elderly. All these symptoms are relieved by HORMONE REPLACEMENT THERAPY involving oestrogen and progesterone which is now generally recognized to be of great benefit.

menstrual cycle and **menstruation** the cyclical nature of the reproductive life of a sexually mature female. One OVUM develops and matures within a GRAAFIAN FOLLICLE in one of the ovaries. When mature, the follicle ruptures to release the egg which passes down the FALLOPIAN TUBE to the uterus. The ruptured follicle becomes a temporary ENDOCRINE GLAND called the CORPUS LUTEUM which secretes the HORMONE, PROGESTERONE. Under the influence of progesterone the uterus wall (ENDOMETRIUM), thickens and its blood supply increases in readiness for the implantation of a fertilized egg. If the egg is not fertilized and there is no pregnancy, the thickened endometrium is shed along with a flow of blood through the vagina (menstruation). The usual age at which menstruation starts is 12 to 15 but it can be as early as 10, or as late as 20. The duration varies and can be anything from 2 to 8 days, the whole cycle usually occupying about 29 to 30 days.

mercaptopurine a type of ANTIMETAB-OLITE, CYTOTOXIC drug which prevents the proliferation of malignant cancer cells and is used in the treatment of certain kinds of LEUKAEMIA, and Crohn's disease (a disease of the digestive tract).

mesencephalon otherwise known as the mid-brain which connects the PONS and CEREBELLUM with the *cerebral hemispheres*.

mesentery a double layer of the peritoneal membrane (PERITONEUM) which is attached to the back wall of the abdomen. It supports a number of abdominal organs including the stomach, small intestine, spleen and pancreas and contains associated nerves, lymph and blood vessels.

mesothelioma a malignant tumour of the PLEURA of the chest cavity and also of the PERICARDIUM or PERITONEUM. It is usually associated with exposure to asbestos dust but may arise independently with no known cause. Most mesotheliomas are in sites which render them inoperable, and chemotherapy and radiotherapy are used but often with limited success.

metabolism the sum of all the physical and chemical changes within cells and tissues that maintain life and growth. The breakdown processes which occur are known as *catabolic (catabolism)*, and those which build materials up are called *anabolic (anabolism)*. The term may also be applied to describe one particular set of changes e.g. *protein metabolism*. *Basal metabolism* is the minimum amount of energy required to maintain the body's vital processes e.g. heartbeat and respiration and is usually assessed by means of various measurements taken while a person is at rest.

metacarpal bone one of the five bones of the middle of the hand between the PHALANGES of the fingers and the CARPAL bones of the wrist forming the *metacarpus*. The heads of the metacarpal bones form the knuckles, *see* HAND.

metaplasia an abnormal change which has taken place within a tissue e.g. *myeloid metaplasia* where elements of bone marrow develop within the spleen and liver. Also *squamous metaplasia* which involves a change in the EPITHELIUM lining the BRONCHI of the lungs.

metastasis the process by which a malignant tumour spreads to a distant part of the body, and also refers to the secondary growth that results from this. The spread is accomplished by means of three routes, the blood circulation, lymphatic system and across body cavities.

metatarsal bone one of the five bones in the foot lying between the toes and the TARSAL bones of the ankle, together forming the *metatarsus*. The metatarsal bones are equivalent to the METACARPAL BONES in the hand.

methadone a strong ANALGESIC and narcotic drug resembling morphine which is used in pain relief and as a cough suppressant. Additionally, it is used as a heroin substitute in the treatment of addiction.

methyldopa a drug that is used to reduce high blood pressure especially in pregnancy.

metritis inflammation of the womb.

MHC major histocompatibility complex - a group of genes located on chromosome 6 which code for the HLA antigens.

microbiology the scientific study of microorganisms i.e. those that are too small to be studied with the naked eye. They include viruses and bacteria, some of which are major causes of disease in man and animals.

microcephaly the condition in which there is abnormal smallness of the head compared to the rest of the body, *see* MACROCEPHALY.

microsurgery surgery performed with the aid of an operating microscope using high precision miniaturized instruments. It is routine for some operations on the eye, larynx and ear and increasingly in areas inaccessible to normal surgery e.g. parts of the brain and spinal cord. Microsurgery is also performed in

the rejoining of severed limbs, fingers, toes etc. where very fine suturing of minute blood vessels and nerves is required.

microwave therapy the use of very short wavelength electromagnetic waves in the procedure known as DIATHERMY.

micturition the act of urination.

middle ear *see* EAR.

midwifery the profession devoted to the care of mothers during pregnancy and childbirth and of mothers and babies during the period after delivery. A member of the profession is known as a *midwife*.

migraine a very severe throbbing headache, usually on one side of the head, which is often accompanied by disturbances in vision, nausea and vomiting. Migraine is a common condition and seems to be triggered by any one or several of a number of factors. These include anxiety, fatigue, watching television or video screens, loud noises, flickering lights (e.g. strobe lights) and certain foods such as cheese and chocolate or alcoholic drinks. The cause is unknown but thought to involve constriction followed by dilation of blood vessels in the brain and an outpouring of fluid into surrounding tissues. The attack can last up to 24 hours and treatment is by means of bed rest in a darkened, quiet room and pain-relieving drugs.

miscarriage *see* ABORTION.

mitobronitol a type of drug used in the treatment of leukaemia which prevents the growth of cancer cells.

mitochondrion a tiny rodlike structure, numbers of which are present in the CYTOPLASM of every CELL. *Mito-*

chondria contain enzymes and ATP involved in cell METABOLISM.

mitosis the type of cell division undergone by most body cells by means of which growth and repair of tissues can take place. Mitosis involves the division of a single cell to produce two genetically identical daughter cells each with the full number of chromosomes, *compare* MEIOSIS.

mitral incompetence also known as *mitral regurgitation*, this is the condition in which the MITRAL VALVE of the heart is defective and allows blood to leak back from the left ventricle into the left atrium. It is often caused by rheumatic fever, as a congenital defect or as a result of a heart attack. The left ventricle is forced to work harder and enlarges, but eventually may be unable to cope and this can result in left-sided heart failure. Other symptoms include atrial FIBRILLATION, breathlessness and embolism. Drug treatment and/or surgery to replace the defective valve may be required (*mitral prosthesis*, *see* MITRAL STENOSIS *and* HEART).

mitral stenosis the condition in which the opening between the left atrium and left ventricle is narrowed due to scarring and adhesion of the MITRAL VALVE. This scarring is often caused by rheumatic fever and the symptoms are similar to those of MITRAL INCOMPETENCE, accompanied also by a *diastolic murmur*. It is treated surgically by widening the stenosis (mitral VALVOTOMY) or by valve replacement - *mitral prosthesis*.

mitral valve formerly known as the *bicuspid valve*, this is located between the atrium and ventricle of the left side of the heart attached to the walls at the opening between the two. It has two cusps or flaps and normally allows blood to pass into the ventricle from the atrium, but prevents any back flow.

MMR vaccine a recently-introduced vaccine (1988) which protects against MEASLES, MUMPS and RUBELLA (German measles) and is normally given to children during their second year.

mole a dark-coloured pigmented spot in the skin which is usually brown. It may be flat or raised and may have hair protruding from it. Some types can become malignant, *see* MELANOMA.

monocyte the largest type of white blood cell (leucocyte) with a kidney-shaped nucleus found in the blood and lymph. It ingests foreign bodies such as bacteria and tissue particles.

mononucleosis *see* GLANDULAR FEVER.

monozygotic twins also known as *identical twins*, these are children who are derived from a single fertilized egg.

morbidity the state of being diseased, the *morbidity rate* being expressed as the number of cases of a disease occurring within a particular number of the population.

moribund dying.

morning sickness vomiting and nausea, most common during the first three months of pregnancy.

morphine a narcotic and very strong analgesic drug which is an alkaloid derived from opium. It is used for the relief of severe pain but tolerance and dependence may occur, *see* ADDICTION.

motion sickness or travel sickness,

produces symptoms of vomiting, nausea and headache caused by travel via car, boat or aeroplane. The symptoms are caused by overstimulation of the balance mechanism in the inner ear through numerous changes in position and an inability to rapidly adjust to them. Although unpleasant, the symptoms are generally not serious and a number of drugs are used to alleviate the condition or to try and prevent its onset.

motor nerve a nerve containing motor neurone fibres which carries electrical impulses outwards from the central nervous system to a muscle or gland to bring about a response there.

motor neurone one of the units or fibres of a MOTOR NERVE. An *upper motor neurone* is contained entirely within the central nervous system having its cell body in the brain and its *axon* (a long process) extending into the spinal cord where it SYNAPSES with other neurones. A *lower motor neurone* has its cell body in the spinal cord or brain stem and an axon that runs outwards via a spinal or cranial MOTOR NERVE to an effector muscle or gland, *see* NERVE.

motorneurone disease a disease of unknown cause which most commonly occurs in middle age and is a degenerative condition affecting elements of the central nervous system (i.e. the corticospinal fibres, motor nuclei in the brain stem and the cells of the anterior horn of the spinal cord). It causes increasing paralysis involving nerves and muscles and is ultimately fatal.

mouth the opening which forms the beginning of the alimentary canal and in which food enters the digestive process. The entrance is guarded by the lips behind which lie the upper and lower sets of teeth embedded in the jaw. The roof of the mouth is called the palate, the front part being hard and immobile while behind lies the mobile soft palate. The tongue is situated behind the lower teeth and SALIVARY GLANDS which are present secrete saliva into the mouth through small ducts. Saliva contains the enzyme ptyalin which begins the breakdown of starch while the chewing action of the teeth and manipulation with the tongue reduces the food to a more manageable size so that it can be swallowed.

mucosa another term for MUCOUS MEMBRANE.

mucous membrane a moist membrane which lines many tubes and cavities within the body and is lubricated with MUCUS. The structure of a mucous membrane varies according to its site and they are found, for example, lining the mouth, respiratory, urinary and digestive tracts. Each has a surface EPITHELIUM, a layer containing various cells and glands which secrete mucus. Beneath this lie connective tissue and muscle layers, the *laminae propria* and *muscularis mucosa* respectively, the whole forming a pliable layer.

mucus a slimy substance secreted by MUCOUS MEMBRANES as a lubricant, and composed mainly of glycoproteins of which the chief one is *mucin*. It is a clear viscous fluid which may contain enzymes and has a protective function. It is normally present in small amounts but the quantity increases if inflammation and/or infection is present.

multiple births twins, triplets, quadruplets, quintuplets and sextuplets born to one mother. While naturally-occurring twins are relatively common, other multiple births are normally rare. Their incidence has increased with the advent of *fertility drugs* although often some of the infants do not survive.

multiple sclerosis a disease of the brain and spinal cord which affects the MYELIN sheaths of nerves and disrupts their function. It usually affects people below the age of 40 and its cause is unknown, but is the subject of much research. The disease is characterized by the presence of patches of hardened (sclerotic) connective tissue irregularly scattered through the brain and spinal cord. At first the fatty part of the nerve sheaths breaks down and is absorbed, leaving bare nerve fibres, and then connective tissue is laid down. Symptoms depend upon the site of the patches in the central nervous system and the disease is characterized by periods of progression and remission. However, they include unsteady gait and apparent clumsiness, tremor of the limbs, involuntary eye movements, speech disorders, bladder disfunction and paralysis. The disease can progress very slowly but generally there is a tendency for the paralysis to become more marked.

mumps an infectious disease of childhood usually occurring in those between the ages of 5 to 15, and caused by a virus which produces inflammation of the *parotid salivary glands*. The incubation period is two to three weeks followed by symptoms including feverishness, headache, sore throat and vomiting, before or along with a swelling of the parotid gland on one side of the face. The swelling may be confined to one side or spread to the other side of face and also may go on to include the *submaxillary* and *sublingual salivary glands* beneath the jaw. Generally after a few days the swelling subsides and the child recovers but remains infectious until the glands have returned to normal. The infection may spread to the pancreas and, in 15 to 30% of males, to the testicles. In adult men this infection can cause sterility. More rarely, inflammation in females can affect the ovaries and breasts, and MENINGITIS is another occasional complication, especially in adults. A protective vaccine is now available, *see* MMR.

Munchausen's syndrome a rare mental disorder in which a person tries to obtain hospital treatment for a nonexistent illness. The person is adept at simulating symptoms and may self-induce these or cause self-inflicted injury to add authenticity. The person may end up having unnecessary treatment and operations and is resistant to psychotherapy.

murmur a characteristic sound which can be heard using a STETHOSCOPE, caused by uneven blood flow through the heart or blood vessels when these are diseased or damaged. Heart murmurs can also be present in normal individuals, especially children, without indicating disease. Murmurs are classified as *diastolic* (when the ventricles are relaxed and filling with blood) or *systolic*, when they are contracting.

muscle the contractile tissue of the body which produces movements of various structures both internally and externally. There are three types of muscle: 1. *striated* or *voluntary muscle* which has a striped appearance when viewed under a microscope and is attached to the skeleton. It is called 'voluntary' because it is under the control of the will and produces movements, for example, in the limbs. 2. *smooth* or *involuntary muscle* which has a plain appearance when viewed microscopically and is not under conscious control but is supplied by the autonomic nervous system. Examples are the muscles which supply the digestive and respiratory tracts. 3. *cardiac muscle*, the specialized muscle of the walls of the heart which is composed of a network of branching, elongated fibres which rejoin and interlock, each having a nucleus. It has a striated appearance and where there are junctions between fibres, irregular transverse bands occur known as *intercalated discs*. This muscle is involuntary and contracts and expands rhythmically throughout a person's life. However, rate of heart beat is affected by activity within the vagus nerve.

muscle cramp *see* CRAMP.

muscle relaxants substances or drugs which cause muscles to relax. They are mainly used in anaesthesia to produce relaxation or paralysis of muscles while surgery is being carried out, e.g. tubocurarine and gallamine. Others are administered to counteract muscular spasms, which are a feature of spastic condi-

tions such as PARKINSONISM, e.g. diazepam.

muscular dystrophy also known as *myopathy*, this is any of a group of diseases which involve wasting of muscles and in which an hereditary factor is involved. The disease is classified according to the groups of muscles which it affects and the age of the person involved. The disease usually appears in childhood and causes muscle fibres to degenerate and to be replaced by fatty and fibrous tissue. The affected muscles eventually lose all power of contraction causing great disability and affected children are prone to chest and other infections which may prove fatal in their weakened state. The cause of the disease is not entirely understood but the commonest form, *Duchenne muscular dystrophy*, is sex-linked and recessive. Hence it nearly always affects boys, with the mother as a carrier, and appears in very early childhood, *see also* SEX-LINKED DISORDERS.

mutation a change which takes place in the DNA, (the genetic material) of the CHROMOSOMES of a cell which is normally a rare event. The change may involve the structure or number of whole chromosomes or take place at one GENE site. Mutations are caused by faulty replication of the cell's genetic material at cell division. If normal body (*somatic*) cells are involved there may be a growth of altered cells or a tumour, or these may be attacked and destroyed by the immune system. In any event, this type of mutation cannot be passed on - if the sex cells (ova or sperm) are involved in the mutation, the alteration may be passed on to the offspring producing a changed characteristic.

mutism the refusal or inability to speak which may result from brain damage or psychological factors. Speechlessness is most common in those who have been born deaf (deaf-mutism).

myalgia pain in a muscle.

myalgic encephalomyelitis (ME) a disorder characterized by muscular pain, fatigue, general depression and loss of memory and concentration. The cause is not understood, but seems to follow on from viral infections such as influenza, hence it is also called post-viral fatigue syndrome. Recovery may be prolonged and there is no specific treatment.

myasthenia gravis a serious and chronic condition of uncertain cause which may be an autoimmune disease. It is more common among young people, especially women (men tend to be affected over 40). Rest and avoidance of unnecessary exertion is essential to conserve muscle strength as there is a reduction in the ability of the neurotransmitter, ACETYLCHOLINE, to effect muscle contraction. There is a weakening which affects skeletal muscles and those for breathing and swallowing etc. However, there is little wasting of the muscles themselves. It seems the body produces antibodies which interfere with the acetylcholine receptors in the muscle, and that the THYMUS GLAND may be the original source of these receptors. Surgical removal of the thymus gland is one treatment. Other treatment is by means of drugs, e.g. Pyridodstig-

mine, which inhibit the activity of the enzyme *cholinesterase* which destroys excess acetylcholine. Other *immunosuppressive* drugs are used to suppress production of the antibodies which interfere with the receptors.

mycosis any disease which is caused by fungi, e.g. THRUSH and RINGWORM.

myelin a sheath of phospholipid and protein that surrounds the axons of some NEURONS. It is formed by specialized cells known as *Schwann cells*, each of which encloses the axon in concentric folds of its cell membrane. These folds then condense to form myelin, the neuron then being described as *myelinated*. Schwann cells produce myelin at regular intervals along the length of the axon and electrical impulses pass more rapidly along myelinated nerve fibres than along non-myelinated ones.

myelitis 1. any inflammatory condition of the spinal cord such as often occurs in MULTIPLE SCLEROSIS. 2. bone marrow inflammation, *see* OSTEOMYELITIS.

myelofibrosis a disease, the cause of which is unknown, in which FIBROSIS takes place within the bone marrow, and many immature red and white blood cells appear in the circulation because of the resultant anaemia. There is an enlargement of the SPLEEN, and blood-producing (myeloid) tissue is abnormally found both here and in the liver.

myelography a specialized X-ray technique involving the injection of a radio-opaque dye into the central canal of the spinal cord in order to distinguish the presence of disease. The X-rays are called *myelograms*.

myeloid means like or relating to bone marrow or, like a *myelocyte*. This is a cell which is an immature type of granulocyte responsible for the production of white blood cells.

myeloma a malignant disease of the bone marrow in which tumours are present in more than one bone at the same time. The bones may show 'holes' when X-rayed due to typical deposits, and certain abnormal proteins may be present in the blood and urine. Treatment is by chemotherapy and radiotherapy. *Myelomatosis* is the production of myeloma which is usually fatal.

myocardial infarction *see* CORONARY THROMBOSIS.

myocarditis inflammation of the muscle in the wall of the heart.

myocardium the middle of the three layers of the HEART wall which is the thick, muscular area. The outer layer is the *epicardium* (forming part of the *pericardium*) and the inner *endocardium*.

myoglobin an iron-containing pigment which is similar to HAEMOGLOBIN, and occurs in muscle cells. It binds oxygen from haemoglobin and releases it in the muscle cells.

myoma a benign tumour in muscle, often in the WOMB.

myomectomy surgical removal of FIBROIDS from the muscular wall of the WOMB (UTERUS).

myometrium the muscular tissue of the WOMB, composed of smooth muscle and surrounding the ENDOMETRIUM. Its contractions are influenced by the presence of certain hormones and are especially strong during LABOUR.

myopathy *see* MUSCULAR DYSTROPHY.

myopia short-sightedness corrected by wearing spectacles with concave lenses.

myxoedema a disease caused by under-activity of the thyroid gland (HYPOTHYROIDISM). There is a characteristic development of a dry, coarse skin and swelling of subcutaneous tissue. There is intellectual impairment with slow speech and mental dullness, lethargy, muscle pain, weight gain and constipation. The hair thins and there may be increased sensitivity to cold. As the symptoms are caused by the deficiency of thyroid hormones, treatment consists of giving THYROXINE in suitable amounts.

N

naevus *see* BIRTHMARK.

narcolepsy a condition whereby a person has a tendency to fall asleep a few times per day for several minutes or hours. The attacks may occur when in quiet surroundings or may be induced by laughter and the person may be woken easily. It is thought that it may be an immune-related disease and lasts for life.

narcosis a state induced by narcotic drugs in which a person is completely unconscious or nearly so but can respond a little to stimuli. It is due to the depressant action of the drugs on the body.

narcotic a drug that leads to a stupor and complete loss of awareness. In particular opiates derived from morphine or produced synthetically produce various conditions: deep sleep, euphoria, mood changes and mental confusion. In addition, respiration and the cough reflex are depressed and muscle spasms may be produced. Because of the dependence resulting from the use of morphine-like compounds, they have largely been replaced for sleeping drugs.

nasal cavity one of two cavities in the nose, divided by a SEPTUM, which lie between the roof of the mouth and the floor of the cranium.

nasogastric tube a small diameter tube passed through the nose into the stomach for purposes of introducing food or drugs or removing fluid (ASPIRATION).

nausea a feeling of being about to vomit. It may be due to motion sickness, early pregnancy, pain, food poisoning or a virus.

nebula a slight opacity or scar of the cornea that does not obstruct vision but may create a haziness. Also an oily substance applied in a fine spray.

nebulizer a device for producing a fine spray. Many inhaled drugs are administered in this way, and it is an effective method of delivering a concentrated form of medication e.g. bronchodilators.

necrosis death of tissue in a localized area or organ, caused by disease, injury or loss of blood supply.

neomycin an antibiotic, usually applied as a cream and which is effective against a wide spectrum of bacteria. Its main use is as a skin treatment.

neonatal term meaning relating to the first 28 days of life.

neoplasm a new and abnormal growth of cells i.e. a tumour, which may be benign or malignant.

nephrectomy surgical removal of all (*radical*) or part of the kidney (*partial*). It may be necessary to remove a tumour (in which case the surrounding fat and adrenal gland will probably also be removed) or to drain an ABSCESS.

nephritis inflammation of the KIDNEY, which may be due to one of several causes. Types of nephritis include glomerulonephritis (when the glomerulus is affected), acute nephritis, hereditary nephritis, etc.

nephron *see* KIDNEY.

nerve a bundle of nerve fibres comprising NEURONS and glial (supporting) cells (*see* GLIA), all contained in a fibrous sheath, the perineurium. Motor nerves carry (efferent) impulses in motor neurons from the brain (or spinal cord) to muscles or glands and a sensory nerve carries (afferent) impulses in sensory neurons from sensory organs to the brain or spinal cord. Most large nerves are mixed nerves containing both motor and sensory nerves.

nerve block (*or* **conduction anaesthesia**) the technique of blocking sensory nerves sending pain impulses to the brain, thus creating anaesthesia in that part of the body. It is achieved by injecting the tissue around a nerve with local anaesthetic (e.g. LIGNOCAINE) to permit minor operations.

nerve injury nerves may be injured by being severed, pressure may damage a nerve directly or push it against a bone. Damage to a sensory nerve results in a lack of or lessening in sensation, while paralysis of muscles will result from damage to the associated motor nerve.

nerve impulse the transmission of information along a nerve fibre by electrical activity which has its basis in the formation of chemical substances and the generation of the *action potential*. This is a change in electrical potential across the cell membrane (between inside and outside) of an axon (nerve cell) as an impulse moves along.

nervous system the complete system of tissues and cells including NERVES, NEURONS, SYNAPSES and receptors (a special cell sensitive to a particular stimulus which then sends an impulse through the nervous system). The nervous system operates through the transmission of impulses (*see* NERVE IMPULSE) that are conducted rapidly to and from muscles, organs etc. It consists of the central nervous system (brain and spinal cord) and the peripheral nervous system that includes the cranial and spinal nerves (*see* AUTONOMIC NERVOUS SYSTEM).

neuralgia strictly, pain in some part or the whole of a nerve (without any physical change in the nerve) but used more widely to encompass pain following the course of a nerve or its branches, whatever the cause. Neuralgia often occurs at the same time each day and is frequently an agonizing pain. It occurs in several forms and is named accordingly, e.g. SCIATICA, trigeminal neuralgia (affecting the face, *see* TRIGEMINAL NERVE) and intercostal neuralgia (affecting the ribs).

neuritis inflammation of a nerve or nerves which may be due to inflammation from nearby tissues, or a more general condition in which the nerve fibres degenerate. This latter condition (*polyneuritis*) is due to a systemic poison such as alcohol or long-term exposure to solvents such as naphtha.

neuroendocrine system one of a number of dual control systems regulating bodily functions through the action of nerves and hormones.

neuroglia the fine web of tissues that support nerve fibres (*see* GLIA).

neurohormone a hormone that is secreted by the nerve endings of specialized nerve cells (i.e. neurosecretory cells) and not by an endocrine gland. They are secreted into the bloodstream or directly into the target tissue. Included are NORADRENALINE and VASOPRESSIN (produced in the HYPOTHALAMUS and secreted by the pituitary gland-active in the control of water reabsorption in the kidneys).

neuroleptic any drug that induces neurolepsis, that is, reduced activity, some indifference to the surroundings and possibly sleep. They are used to quieten disturbed patients suffering from delirium, brain damage or behavioural disturbances.

neurology the subdiscipline of medicine that involves the study of the brain, spinal cord and peripheral nerves, their diseases and conditions and the treatment of those conditions.

neuromuscular blockade the blocking of impulses at the NEUROMUSCULAR JUNCTION to paralyse a part of the body for surgery (*see also* NERVE BLOCK).

neuromuscular junction the area of membrane between a muscle cell and a motor NEURON forming a SYNAPSE between the two. Nerve impulses travel down the neuron and each releases ACETYLCHOLINE which depolarizes the enlarged end of the neuron (the motor end plate) slightly. These small depolarization are totalled until a threshold of -50mV is reached and this results in the production of an ACTION POTENTIAL that crosses the synapse into the muscle fibre producing a muscle contraction.

neuron a nerve cell, vital in the transmission of impulses. Each cell has an enlarged portion (the cell body) from which extends the long, thin axon for carrying impulses away. Shorter, more numerous dendrites receive impulses. The transmission of impulses is faster in axons that are covered in a sheath of MYELIN.

neuropathy any disease that affects the peripheral nerves, whether singly (mononeuropathy) or more generally (polyneuropathy). The symptoms depend upon the type and the nerves affected.

neurosurgery surgical treatment of the brain, spinal cord or nerves, including dealing with head injuries, intracranial pressure, haemorrhages, infections and the treatment of tumours.

neurotransmitter one of several chemical substances released in minute quantities by axon tips into the SYNAPSE to enable a nerve impulse to cross. It diffuses across the space and may depolarize the opposite membrane allowing the production of an action potential (*see* NERVE IMPULSE). Outside the central nervous system ACETYLCHOLINE is a major neurotransmitter, and NORADRENALINE is released in the SYMPATHETIC NERVOUS SYSTEM. Acetylcholine and noradrenaline also operate within the central nervous system as does DOPAMINE, amongst others.

night blindness (nyctalopia) poor vision in dim light or at night due to a deficiency within the cells responsible for such vision (*see* ROD). The cause may be a lack of VITAMIN A in the diet or a congenital defect.

nitrous oxide formerly called laughing gas, a colourless gas used for anaesthesia over short periods. Longer effects require its use with oxygen and it may be used as a 'carrier' for stronger anaesthetics.

non-steroidal anti-inflammatory drugs (NSAID) a large group of drugs used to relieve pain, and also inhibit inflammation. They are used for conditions such as rheumatoid arthritis, sprains etc. and include aspirin. The main side-effect is gastric ulcer or haemorrhage but the synthesis of new compounds has led to some with milder side-effects.

noradrenaline (norepinephrine in US) a NEUROTRANSMITTER of the SYMPATHETIC NERVOUS SYSTEM secreted by nerve endings and also the adrenal glands. It is similar to ADRENALINE in structure and function. It increases blood pressure by constricting the vessel, slows the heartbeat, increases breathing both in rate and depth.

nose the olfactory organ and also a pathway for air entering the body, by which route it is warmed, filtered and moistened before passing into the lungs. The 'external' nose leads to the NASAL CAVITY which has a mucous membrane with olfactory cells.

notifiable diseases diseases that must be reported to the health authorities to enable rapid control and monitoring to be undertaken. The list varies between countries but in the U.K. includes acute poliomyelitis, AIDS, cholera, dysentery, food poisoning, measles, meningitis, rabies, rubella, scarlet fever, smallpox, tetanus, typhoid fever, viral hepatitis and whooping cough.

nuclear magnetic resonance an analytical technique based upon the absorption of electromagnetic radiation over specific frequencies for those nuclei that spin about their own axes. The result is a change in orientation of the nuclei and certain elements are particularly susceptible (hydrogen, fluorine and phosphorus). The technique has been developed into a medical imaging tool which can create an image of soft tissues in any part of the body.

nucleic acid a linear molecule that occurs in two forms: DNA (deoxyribonucleic acid) and RNA (ribonucleic acid), composed of four NUCLEOTIDES. DNA is the major part of CHROMOSOMES in the cell nucleus while RNA is found outside the nucleus and is involved in protein synthesis.

nucleotide the basic molecular building block of the nucleic acids RNA and DNA. A nucleotide comprises a five-carbon sugar molecule with a phosphate group and an organic base. The organic base can be a *purine*, e.g. adenine and guanine or a *pyrimidine* e.g. cytosine and thymine as in DNA. In RNA uracil replaces thymine.

nucleus the large organelle (a membrane-bounded cell constituent) that contains the DNA. Unless it is dividing a nucleolus with RNA is present. During cell division the DNA, which is normally dispersed with protein (as chromatin), forms visible CHROMOSOMES.

O

obesity the accumulation of excess fat in the body, mainly in the subcutaneous tissues, caused by eating more food than is necessary to produce the required energy for each day's activity. The effects of obesity are serious, being associated with increased mortality or cause of illness from cardiovascular disease, diabetes, gall bladder complaints, hernia and many others. Treatment involves a low energy diet but more drastic measures (e.g. stapling of the stomach) may be necessary.

obstetrics the subdiscipline of medicine that deals with pregnancy and childbirth and the period immediately after birth; midwifery.

occipital bone a bone of the SKULL which is shaped like a saucer and forms the back of the cranium and part of its base. Arising from the base of thin bone are two occipital condyles that articulate with the first cervical vertebrae (the atlas) of the spinal column.

occlusion the closing or blocking of an organ or duct. In dentistry it is the way the teeth meet when the jaws are closed.

occult a term meaning not easily seen; not visible to the naked eye.

occupational diseases (or industrial diseases) diseases, specific to a particular occupation, and to which workers in that occupation are prone. There are many lung conditions including: PNEUMOCONIOSIS (from coal mining); SILICOSIS (mining, stone dressing, etc.); ASBESTOSIS; FARMER'S LUNG (from fungal spores), and so on. In addition there are dangers from excessive noise, irritant chemicals, occupations resulting in musculo-skeletal disorders, decompression sickness (*see also* BENDS) radiation and infections from either animals or humans.

oculomotor nerve either of a pair of cranial nerves which are involved in eye movements including movement of the eyeball, and alterations in the size of the pupil and lens.

oedema an accumulation of fluid in the body, possibly beneath the skin or in cavities or organs. With an injury the swelling may be localized or more general as in cases of kidney or heart failure. Fluid can collect in the chest cavity, abdomen or lung (PULMONARY OEDEMA). The causes are numerous, e.g. CIRRHOSIS of the liver, heart or kidney failure, starvation, acute NEPHRITIS, allergies or drugs. To alleviate the symptom, the root cause has to be removed. Subcutaneous oedema commonly occurs in women before menstruation, as swollen legs or ankles, but does subside if the legs are rested in a raised position.

oesophagoscope an instrument for inspecting the oesophagus. It has a light source and can be used to open the tube if narrowed, remove material for biopsy or remove an obstruction.

oesophagus the first part of the ALIMENTARY CANAL lying between the PHARYNX and stomach. The mucous membrane lining produces secretions to lubricate food as it passes and the movement of the food to the stomach is achieved by waves of muscular movement called *peristalsis*.

oestradiol the major female sex hormone. It is produced by the ovary and is responsible for development of the breasts, sexual characteristics and premenstrual uterine changes.

oestrogen one of a group of STEROID hormones secreted mainly by the ovaries and to a lesser extent by the adrenal cortex and placenta. (The testes also produce small amounts). Oestrogens control the female secondary sexual characteristics, i.e. enlargement of the breasts, change in the profile of the pelvic girdle, pubic hair growth and deposition of body fat. High levels are produced at ovulation and with PROGESTERONE they regulate the female reproductive cycle.

Naturally-occurring oestrogens include OESTRADIOL, oestriol and oestrone. Synthetic varieties are used in the contraceptive pill and to treat gynaecological disorders.

olfaction the sense of smell, *see* NOSE.

olfactory nerve one of a pair of sensory nerves for smell. It is the first cranial nerve and comprises many fine threads connecting receptors in the mucous membrane of the olfactory area which pass through holes in the skull, fuse to form one fibre and then pass back to the brain.

oncogene any GENE directly involved in cancer, whether in viruses or in the individual.

oncogenic any factor that causes cancer. This may be an organism, a chemical or some environmental condition. Some viruses are oncogenic and have the result of making a normal cell become a cancer cell.

oncology the subdiscipline of medicine concerned with the study and treatment of tumours, including medical, surgical aspects and their treatment with radiation.

oocyte a cell in the OVARY that undergoes MEIOSIS to produce an OVUM, the female reproductive cell. A newborn female already has primary oocytes, of which only a small number survive to puberty, and even then only a fraction will be ovulated (*see* OVULATION).

operculum a lid, plug or flap. A term used in several areas of medicine e.g. it is a plug of mucus blocking the cervix in a pregnant woman; it is also used in neurology and dentistry.

ophthalmology the branch of medicine dealing with the structure of the eye, its function, associated diseases and treatment.

ophthalmoplegia paralysis of the muscles serving the EYE, which may be internal (affecting the iris and ciliary muscle) or external (those muscles moving the eye itself).

opiate one of several drugs, derived from opium and including morphine and codeine. They act by depressing the central nervous system, thus relieving pain and suppressing coughing. Morphine and heroin, its synthetic derivative, are narcotics.

opium a milky liquid extracted from the unripe seed capsules of the poppy, *Papaver somniferum* which has almost 10% of anhydrous morphine. Opium is a NARCOTIC and ANALGESIC.

opportunistic an infection that is contracted by someone with a lower resistance than usual. This may be due to drugs or another disease such as DIABETES MELLITUS, CANCER or AIDS. In normal circumstances, in a healthy person, the infecting organism would not cause the disease.

optic atrophy a deterioration and wasting of the optic disc due to degeneration of fibres in the optic nerve. It may accompany numerous conditions including DIABETES, ARTERIOSCLEROSIS, GLAUCOMA or may be due to a congenital defect, inflammation or injury, or toxic poisoning from alcohol, lead, etc.

optic chiasma (**optic commissure**) the cross-shaped structure formed from a crossing over of the optic nerves running back from the eyeballs to meet beneath the brain in the midline.

orchidectomy removal of one or both (castration) testes, usually to treat a malignant growth.

orchidopexy the operation performed to bring an undescended testis into the scrotum. It is undertaken well before puberty to ensure normal development subsequently.

organ any distinct and recognizable unit within the body that is composed of two or more types of tissue and that is responsible for a particular function or functions. Examples are the liver, kidney, heart and brain.

orgasm the climax of sexual arousal which in men coincides with ejaculation and comprises a series of involuntary muscle contractions. In women there are irregular contractions of the vagina walls.

orthodontics a part of dentistry dealing with development of the teeth and the treatment of (or prevention of) any disorders.

orthopaedics the subdiscipline of medicine concerned with the study of the skeletal system and the joints, muscles etc. It also covers the treatment of bone damage or disease whether CONGENITAL or acquired.

orthopnoea a severe difficulty in breathing so that a patient cannot lie and has to sleep in a sitting position. It usually only occurs with serious conditions of the heart and lungs.

osmosis the process whereby solvent molecules (usually water) move through a semipermeable membrane to the more concentrated solution. Cell membranes function as semipermeable membranes and osmosis is important in regulating water content in living systems.

ossicle the term for a small bone, of-

ten applied to those of the middle ear, the auditory ossicles (see EAR), that transmit sound to the inner ear from the eardrum.

ossification (or **osteogenesis**) bone formation, which occurs in several stages via special cells called OSTEOBLASTS. COLLAGEN fibres form a network in connective tissue and then a cement of polysaccharide is laid down. Finally, calcium salts are distributed among the cement as tiny crystals. The osteoblasts are enclosed as bone cells (OSTEOCYTES).

osteitis inflammation of bone, caused by damage, infection or bodily disorder. Symptoms include swelling, tenderness, a dull aching sort of pain and redness cover the affected area.

osteoarthritis a form of ARTHRITIS involving joint cartilage with accompanying changes in the associated bone. It usually involves the loss of cartilage and the development of OSTEOPHYTES at the bone margins. The function of the joint (most often the thumb, knee and hip) is affected and it becomes painful. The condition may be due to overuse, and affects those past middle age. It also may complicate other joint diseases. Treatment usually involves administering ANALGESICS, possibly anti-inflammatory drugs and the use of corrective or replacement surgery.

osteoblast a specialized cell responsible for the formation of bone.

osteochondritis inflammation of bone and cartilage.

osteochondrosis a disease affecting the OSSIFICATION centres of bone in children. It begins with degeneration and NECROSIS but it regenerates and calcifies again.

osteocyte a bone cell formed from an osteoblast that is no longer active and has become embedded in the matrix of the bone.

osteogenesis imperfecta (brittle bone disease) an hereditary disease which results in the bones being unusually fragile and brittle. It may have associated symptoms, namely, transparent teeth, unusually mobile joints, dwarfism, etc. It may be due to a disorder involving COLLAGEN, but there is little that can be done in treatment.

osteomalacia a softening of the bones, and the adult equivalent of rickets, which is due to a lack of VITAMIN D. This vitamin is obtained from the diet and is produced on exposure to sunlight, and it is necessary for the uptake of calcium from food.

osteomyelitis bone marrow inflammation caused by infection. This may happen after a compound fracture or during bone surgery. It produces pain, swelling and fever and high doses of antibiotics are necessary.

osteophyte bony projections that occur near joints or intervertebral discs where cartilage has degenerated or been destroyed (*see* OSTEOARTHRITIS). Osteophytes may in any case occur with increasing age with or without loss of cartilage.

osteoporosis a loss of bone tissue due to it being resorbed, resulting in bones that become brittle and likely to fracture. It is common in menopausal women and results from long-term steroid therapy. It is also a feature of CUSHING'S SYNDROME. Hormone replacement therapy is a treatment available to women.

osteosarcoma the commonest and most malignant bone tumour that is found most in older children. The femur is usually affected but metastases are common (*see* METASTASIS). It produces pain and swelling and although amputation used to be the standard treatment, surgery is now possible, with replacement of the diseased bone and associated chemotherapy and/or radiotherapy. It remains, nevertheless, a serious cancer with a relatively poor survival rate.

osteosclerosis a condition in which the density of bone tissue increases abnormally. It is due to tumour, infection or poor blood supply and may be due to an abnormality involving osteoclasts, cells that resorb calcified bone.

otitis inflammation of the ear. This may take several forms depending upon the exact location which produces diverse symptoms e.g. inflammation of the inner ear (*otitis interna*), affects balance, causing vertigo and vomiting while *otitis media* is usually a bacterial infection of the middle ear resulting in severe pain, and a fever requiring immediate antibiotic treatment. *Secretory otitis media* is otherwise known as GLUE EAR.

otology the subdiscipline of medicine concerned with the ear, its disorders, diseases and their treatment.

ovarian cyst a sac filled with fluid that develops in the ovary. Most are benign but their size may cause swelling and pressure on other organs. For those cysts that do become malignant, it is possible that its discovery comes too late to allow successful treatment. ULTRASOUND scanning can be adopted to detect tumours at an early stage.

ovariotomy literally cutting into an ovary, but more generally used for surgical removal of an ovary or an ovarian tumour.

ovary the reproductive organ of females which produces eggs (ova) and hormones (mainly OESTROGEN and PROGESTERONE). There are two ovaries, each the size of an almond, on either side of the uterus and each contains numerous Graafian FOLLICLES in which the eggs develop. At OVULATION an egg is released from a follicle. The follicles secrete oestrogen and progesterone which regulate the menstrual cycle and the uterus during pregnancy.

ovulation the release of an egg from an OVARY (i.e. from a mature Graafian follicle) which then moves down the FALLOPIAN TUBE to the uterus. Ovulation is brought about by secretion of *luteinizing hormone* secreted by the anterior PITUITARY GLAND.

ovum (*plural* **ova**) the mature, unfertilized female reproductive cell which is roughly spherical with an outer membrane and a single nucleus.

oxytocin a hormone from the PITUITARY GLAND that causes the uterus to contract during LABOUR and prompts lactation due to contraction of muscle fibres in the milk ducts of the breasts.

P

pacemaker the part of the heart that regulates the beat - the SINOATRIAL NODE. Also, in patients with a HEART BLOCK, a device inserted into the body to maintain a normal heart rate. There are different types of pacemaker, some being permanent, others temporary; some stimulate the beat while others are activated only when the natural rate of the heart falls below a certain level.

paediatrics the branch of medicine that deals with children.

paedophilia an abnormal sexual attraction to children.

Paget's disease (of bone) otherwise known as *osteitis deformans*. A chronic bone disease, particularly of the long bones, skull and spine, which results in the bones becoming thickened, disorganized and also soft, causing them to bend. The cause is unknown and although there is also no cure, good results are being obtained with CALCITONIN. The main symptom is pain.

palate the roof of the mouth, that separates the cavity of the mouth below from that of the nose above. It consists of the *hard* and *soft* palate. The hard palate is located at the front of the mouth and is a bony plate covered by mucous membrane. The soft palate is a muscular layer also covered by mucous membrane. The moveable soft palate is important in the production of sounds and speech.

palliative a medicine or treatment that is given to effect some relief from symptoms, if only temporarily, but does not cure the ailment.

palpation examination of the surface of the body by carefully feeling with hands and fingertips. It is often possible to distinguish between solid lumps or swelling and cystic swellings.

palpitation when the heart beats noticeably or irregularly and the person becomes aware of it. The heartbeat is not normally noticed but with fear, emotion or exercise it may be felt, unpleasantly so. Palpitations may also be due to neuroses, ARRHYTHMIA, heart disease and a common cause is too much tea, coffee, alcohol or smoking. Where an excess is the cause (tea, coffee etc.) this can be eliminated. For disease-associated palpitations, drugs can be used for control.

pancreas a gland with both ENDOCRINE and exocrine functions. It is located between the DUODENUM and SPLEEN, behind the stomach, and is about 15cm long. There are two types of cells producing secretions, the *acini* which produce pancreatic juice which goes to the intestine via a system of ducts. This contains an alkaline mixture of salt and enzymes - trypsin and chymotrypsin to digest proteins, amylase to break down starch and lipase to aid digestion of fats. The second cell types are in the ISLETS OF LANGERHANS and these pro-

duce two hormones, INSULIN and GLU-CAGON, secreted directly into the blood for control of sugar levels (*see also* DIABETES MELLITUS, HYPO- and HYPERGLYCAEMIA).

pancreatectomy surgical removal of the PANCREAS (or part of it) to deal with tumours or chronic PANCREATI-TIS. After *total* or *subtotal* pancreatectomy (where all or almost all is removed) the pancreatic secretions to aid digestion and control blood sugar have to be administered.

pancreatitis inflammation of the PAN-CREAS, occurring in several forms, but often associated with gallstones or alcoholism. Any bout of the condition that interferes with the function of the pancreas may lead to DIA-BETES and MALABSORPTION.

pandemic an epidemic that is so widely spread that it affects large numbers of people in a country or countries.

Papanicolaou test (Pap test) another name for a CERVICAL SMEAR.

papilla any small protuberance such as the papillae on the tongue.

papilloma usually benign growths on the skin surface or mucous membrane e.g. WARTS.

paracentesis the procedure of tapping or taking off (excess) fluid from the body by means of a hollow needle or CANNULA.

paracetamol a drug that has analgesic effects and also reduces fever. It is taken for mild pain (headache, etc.). It may cause digestive problems and large doses are very dangerous. Excessive doses can produce liver failure, causing progressive NECROSIS in a matter of days and very large doses are fatal. In the early stages of poisoning the stomach can be washed out and drugs administered to protect the liver.

parainfluenza viruses a group of viruses that cause respiratory tract infections with usually mild influenza-like symptoms. Infants and young children seem to be affected most. There are four types of the virus, virulent at different times of the year.

paralysis muscle weakness or total loss of muscle movement which varies depending upon the causal disease and its effect on the brain. Various descriptive terms are used to qualify the parts of the body affected, thus hemiplegia affects one side of the body (*see also* DIPLEGIA, PARAPLEGIA, QUADRIPLEGIA). Paralysis is really a symptom of another condition or disease e.g. brain disease such as a cerebral haemorrhage or THROMBOSIS causing hemiplegia; disease or injury of the spinal cord leading to paraplegia; and POLIOMYELITIS (infantile paralysis). In addition there is the paralysis associated with MOTOR NEURONE DISEASE.

paraphimosis constriction of the penis due to retraction of an abnormally tight foreskin which contracts on the penis behind the glans, and cannot be easily moved. Swelling and pain may be caused and usually circumcision is necessary to prevent a recurrence.

paraplegia PARALYSIS of the legs. It may be caused by injury or disease of the spinal cord and often bladder and rectum are also affected.

parasite any organism that obtains its nutrients by living in or on the body of another organism (the *host*).

Parasites in humans include worms, viruses, fungi, etc.

parasympathetic nervous system one of the two parts of the AUTONOMIC NERVOUS SYSTEM that acts antagonistically with the SYMPATHETIC NERVOUS SYSTEM. The parasympathetic nerves originate from the brain and lower portion of the spinal cord (sacral region). The AXONS of this system tend to be longer than sympathetic nerves and SYNAPSES with other neurons are close to the target organ. The parasympathetic system contracts the bladder, decreases heart rate, stimulates the sex organs, promotes digestion, etc.

parathyroidectomy removal of the PARATHYROID GLANDS, usually in treatment of hyperparathyroidism (hyperactivity of one or all of the glands).

parathyroid glands four small glands located behind or within the thyroid gland, that control the metabolism of calcium and phosphorus (as phosphate) in the body. The hormone responsible, parathormone (or simply parathyroid hormone) is produced and released by the glands. A deficiency of the hormone leads to lower levels of calcium in the blood with a relative increase in phosphorus. This produces tetany, a condition involving muscular spasms, which can be treated by injection. This is also known as *hypoparathyroidism* and is often due to removal or injury of the glands during thyroidectomy. If the hormone is at high levels calcium is transferred from bones to the blood, causing weakness and susceptibility to breaks.

paratyphoid fever a bacterial infection caused by *Salmonella paratyphi A, B* or *C*. Symptoms resemble those of typhoid fever and include diarrhoea, a rash and mild fever. It can be treated with antibiotics and temporary immunity against the *A* and *B* form is gained by vaccination with TAB vaccine.

parenteral nutrition provision of food by any means other than by the mouth. For patients with burns, renal failure etc. or after major surgery, this mode of feeding may be necessary and is accomplished intravenously. Protein, fat and carbohydrate can all be delivered as special solutions containing all the essential compounds. The main hazard of such a system is the risk of infection and reactions to the solutions introduced e.g. HYPERGLYCAEMIA can result.

parkinsonism a progressive condition occurring in mid to late life which results in a rigidity of muscles affecting the voice and face rather than those in the limbs. A tremor also develops possibly in one hand initially and then spreading to other limbs and it appears most pronounced when sitting. The disease is usually due to a deficiency in the NEUROTRANSMITTER dopamine, due to degeneration of the basal ganglia of the brain (*see* BASAL GANGLION). There is no cure available, but a number of drugs are able, to varying degrees, to control the condition.

parotid gland one of a pair of salivary glands situated in front of each ear and opening inside the cheek near the second last molar of the upper jaw.

parotitis inflammation of the PAROTID GLAND, which as epidemic or infectious parotitis is called MUMPS.

paroxysm a sudden attack. A term used especially about convulsions.

parturition *see* LABOUR.

patch test a test undertaken to identify the substances causing a person's allergy. Different allergens are placed in very small amounts on the skin. A red flare with swelling will develop if the person is allergic. This commonly happens within 15 minutes but may take up to 72 hours.

patella the kneecap. An almost flat bone, shaped somewhat like an oyster shell, that lies in front of the knee in the tendon of the thigh muscle.

patellar reflex *see* REFLEX ACTION.

pathogen the term applied to an organism that causes disease. Most pathogens affecting humans are bacteria and viruses.

pathology the study of the causes, characteristics and effects of disease on the body by examining samples of body fluids and products whether from a living patient or at autopsy.

pectoral the descriptive term for anything relating to the chest.

pectoral girdle (or shoulder girdle) the skeletal structure to which the bones of the upper limbs are attached. It is composed of two shoulder blades (SCAPULAe) and two collar bones (CLAVICLES) attached to the vertebral column and breastbone (sternum) respectively.

pedicle a narrow roll of skin by which a piece of skin for grafting is attached. It is used when it is not possible to place an independent graft on the site, perhaps because of poor blood supply. Also the term for a narrow neck of tissue connecting a tumour to its tissue of origin.

pediculosis a deficiency disease

caused by a lack of nicotinic acid, part of the VITAMIN B complex. It occurs when the diet is based on maize (rather than wheat) with an associated lack of first-class protein (meat and milk). The reason is that although maize contains nicotinic acid it is in an unusable form and also it does not contain the amino acid tryptophan which the body can use to produce nicotinic acid. The symptoms are dermatitis, diarrhoea and depression.

pelvic girdle (or hip girdle) the skeletal structure to which the bones of the lower limbs are attached. It is made up of the two hip bones, each comprising the ilium, pubis and ischium, fused together.

pelvic inflammatory disease an acute or chronic infection of the UTERUS, ovaries or FALLOPIAN TUBES. It is due to infection elsewhere e.g. the appendix, which spreads or as infection carried by the blood. It produces severe abdominal pain which usually responds to antibiotics but surgery may sometimes be necessary to remove diseased tissue.

pelvis the skeletal structure formed by the hip bones, sacrum and coccyx and which connects with the spine and legs. The female pelvis is shallower and the ilia are wider apart and there are certain angular differences to the male, all of which relate to childbearing. The pelvis is a point of contact for the muscles of the legs and it partially envelops the bladder and rectum. In males it also includes the prostate gland and seminal vesicles while in females it contains the womb and ovaries (*see individual entries*).

penicillin the antibiotic derived from the mould *Penicillium notatum* which grows naturally on decaying fruit, bread or cheese. The genus used for production of the drug is *P. chrysogenum.* Penicillin is active against a large range of bacteria and it is nontoxic. It is usually given by injection but can be taken orally. There are many semi-synthetic penicillins acting in different ways including Ampicillin and Propicillin. Some patients are allergic to penicillin but there tend to be very few serious side-effects.

penis the male organ through which the URETHRA passes, carrying urine or semen. It is made up of tissue that is filled with blood during sexual arousal, producing an erection which enables penetration of the vagina and ejaculation of semen. The glans is the end part normally covered by the FORESKIN (prepuce).

peptic ulcer an ulcer in the stomach (GASTRIC ULCER), oesophagus, duodenum (DUODENAL ULCER), or JEJUNUM. It is caused by a break in the mucosal lining due to the action of acid and pepsin (an enzyme active in protein breakdown) either because of their high concentrations or due to other factors affecting the mucosal protective mechanisms.

percussion the diagnostic aid which involves tapping parts of the body (particularly on back and chest) with the fingers to produce a vibration and note-like sound. The sound produced gives an indication of abnormal enlargement of organs, and the presence of fluid in the lungs.

perforation when a hole forms in a hollow organ, tissue or tube, e.g. the stomach, eardrum etc. In particular, it is a serious development of an ulcer in the stomach or bowels because on perforation the intestine contents, with bacteria, enter the peritoneal (*see* PERITONEUM) cavity causing PERITONITIS. This is accompanied by severe pain and shock and usually corrective surgery is required.

pericarditis inflammation of the PERICARDIUM. It may be due to URAEMIA, cancer or viral infection and produces fever, chest pain and possible accumulation of fluid.

pericardium the smooth membrane surrounding the heart. The outer *fibrous* part covers the heart and is connected to the large vessels coming out of the heart. The inner *serous* part is a closed SEROUS MEMBRANE attached both to the fibrous pericardium and the heart wall. Some fluid in the resulting sac enables smooth movement as the heart beats.

perinatal mortality foetal deaths after week 28 of pregnancy and newborn deaths during the first week or two of life. The main causes of perinatal mortality are brain injuries during birth, congenital defects and lack of oxygen in the final stages of pregnancy (called *antepartum anoxia*). Perinatal *deaths* are due to complications involving the placenta, congenital defects and birth asphyxia.

perineum the area of the body between anus and urethral opening.

periodontal descriptive term relating to the tissues surrounding the teeth.

peripheral nervous system those parts of the nervous system excluding the central nervous system (brain and spinal cord). It comprises the afferent (sensory) and efferent (motor) cells which include 12 pairs of cranial nerves and 31 pairs of spinal nerves. The motor nervous system then comprises the somatic nervous system carrying impulses to the skeletal muscles, and the autonomic nervous system which is further divided into the sympathetic and the parasympathetic nervous system (*see individual entries*).

peripheral neuritis inflammation of the nerves of the peripheral system.

peritoneum the SEROUS MEMBRANE that lines the abdominal cavity. That lining the abdomen walls is the *parietal* peritoneum while the *visceral* peritoneum covers the organs. The folds of peritoneum from one organ to another are given special names, e.g. MESENTERY. Both are continuous and form a closed sac at the back of the abdomen in the male, while in the female there is an opening from the Fallopian tube on either side.

peritonitis inflammation of the peritoneum. It may be caused by a primary infection due to bacteria in the bloodstream (e.g. tuberculous peritonitis) resulting in pain and swelling, fever and weight loss. Secondary infection results from entry into the abdominal cavity of bacteria and irritants (e.g. digestive juices) from a perforated or ruptured organ e.g. duodenum or stomach. This produces severe pain and shock and surgery is often necessary.

pernicious anaemia a type of ANAEMIA due to VITAMIN B_{12} deficiency which results from dietary lack or the failure to produce the substance that enables B_{12} to be absorbed from the bowel. This in turn results in a lack of red blood cell production and

MEGALOBLASTS in the bone marrow. The condition is easily treated by regular injections of the vitamin.

perspiration (*or* **sweat**) the excretion from millions of tiny sweat glands in the skin. Sweat that evaporates from the skin immediately is *insensible*, while that forming drops is *sensible perspiration*. Sweat is produced in two types of sweat glands. The *eccrine* glands are found mainly on the soles of the feet and palms of the hands. The *apocrine* glands are in the armpits, around the anus and genitalia and sweat is produced in response to stimuli such as fear and sexual arousal. The major function of sweating, however, is the regulation of body temperature.

Perthes' disease a hip condition in children between the ages of four and ten, and which is self-healing. Due to OSTEOCHONDROSIS of the EPIPHYSIS of the femur a limp is developed with associated pain. Rest is essential as is traction, until the pain subsides and then a special splint is fitted to permit walking until the condition is fully healed.

pertussis *see* WHOOPING COUGH.

pessary an instrument that fits into the vagina to treat a PROLAPSE. Also a soft solid that is shaped for insertion into the vagina and contains drugs for some gynaecological disorder (also used for inducing labour).

pethidine a drug with ANALGESIC and mild sedative action for relief of moderate pain. It may be given by mouth or injection but side-effects include nausea, dizziness and dry mouth, and also prolonged use may create dependence.

petit mal the lesser type of epileptic

seizure which is IDIOPATHIC. It consists of brief periods (seconds) of unconsciousness when the eyes stare blankly but posture is maintained. Children suffering frequently may have learning difficulties but the condition may disappear in adult life.

phagocytosis *see* LEUCOCYTE.

phalanges (*singular* **phalanx**) the bones of the digits (fingers and toes) which number fourteen in each hand and foot. The thumb and big toe comprise two while all the other digits have three phalanges.

phallus penis, or a penis-like object. Also the term used for the embryonic penis before the final development of the urethral duct.

phantom limb the feeling that a limb or part of a limb is still attached to the body after it has been amputated. This is probably due to stimulation of the severed nerves and usually wears off with time.

pharmaceutical relating to pharmacy or drugs.

pharmacist a trained, qualified and registered person who is authorized to keep and dispense medicines.

pharmacology the branch of medicine concerning the preparation, properties, uses and effects of drugs.

pharmacy the preparation of drugs (and their dispensing); or the place where this function is undertaken.

pharyngectomy surgical excision of part of the pharynx.

pharyngitis inflammation of the PHARYNX and therefore throat, commonly due to a virus, and resulting in a sore throat. It is often associated with TONSILLITIS.

pharynx the region extending from the beginning of the oesophagus up to the base of the skull at the cavity into which nose and mouth open. It is muscular, with a mucous membrane and acts as the route for both food (to the oesophagus) and air (to the larynx). The EUSTACHIAN TUBES open from the upper part of the pharynx.

phenobarbitone a very widely used BARBITURATE. It can be given orally or by injection and is taken as an anticonvulsant in epilepsy and to treat insomnia or anxiety. It may produce drowsiness and some skin reactions and continued use should be avoided, lest dependence ensue.

phenotype the detectable, observable characteristics of an individual that are determined by the interaction of his GENES (genotype) and the environment in which he develops. The expression of the dominant gene masks the presence of a recessive one, as only the expressed gene affects the phenotype.

phenyl ketonuria a genetic disorder that results in the deficiency of an ENZYME that converts phenylalanine, an ESSENTIAL AMINO ACID, to tyrosine. Children can be severely mentally retarded by an excess of phenylalanine in the blood damaging the nervous system. The responsible gene is recessive therefore the condition occurs only if both parents are carriers. However, there is a test for newborn infants (the Guthrie test) that ensures the condition can be detected and the diet can be modified to avoid phenylalanine and thus any brain damage.

phial a small glass bottle-like receptacle for storing medicines.

phimosis a condition in which the edge of the FORESKIN is narrowed and

cannot be drawn back over the glans of the PENIS. To avoid inflammation and an exacerbation of the problem, circumcision may be necessary.

phlebectomy removal of a vein, or part of a vein, sometimes undertaken in the treatment of VARICOSE VEINS.

phlebitis inflammation of a vein. This commonly occurs as a complication of VARICOSE VEINS, producing pain and a hot feeling around the vein, with possible THROMBOSIS development. Drugs and elastic support are used in treatment.

phlebothrombosis the obstruction of a vein by a blood clot, common in the deep veins of the leg (in particular the calf) and resulting from heart failure, pregnancy, injury and surgery, which may change the clotting factors in the blood. The affected leg may swell and there is the danger that the clot may move, creating a PULMONARY EMBOLISM. Large clots may be removed surgically, otherwise the treatment involves anticoagulant drugs and exercise.

phlebotomy the opening of a vein, or its puncture, to remove blood or to infuse fluids.

phlegm a general térm (non-medical) for sputum, mucus.

phobia an anxiety disorder and irrational fear of certain objects, animals, situations, events, etc. Avoiding the situation can lead to significant disruption, restriction of normal life or even suffering.

phonation the production of speech sounds.

photophobia an atypical sensitivity to light. Exposure produces discomfort and actions to evade the light source. The condition may be associated with medications, or migraine, meningitis, etc.

phrenic nerve the nerve to the muscles of the DIAPHRAGM, arising from the 3rd, 4th and 5th cervical spinal nerves.

physical concerning the body as opposed to the mind.

physician a registered medical practitioner who deals with non-surgical practice.

physiology the study of the functions of and processes within the body and its various organs.

physiotherapy the use of physical methods to help healing. It may involve exercise, massage and manipulation, heat treatment and the use of light and ultraviolet radiation, etc.

pia mater *see* BRAIN and MENINGES.

pigment an organic colouring agent e.g. the blood pigment HAEMOGLOBIN, BILE pigments, rhodopsin (found in the RODS of the RETINA) and MELANIN.

piles *see* HAEMORRHOIDS.

pilus a hair or structure like a hair.

pituitary gland (*or* **hypophysis**) a small, but very important endocrine gland at the base of the HYPOTHALAMUS. It has two lobes, the anterior *adenohypophysis* and the posterior *neurohypophysis*. The pituitary secretes hormones that control many functions and is itself controlled by hormonal secretions from the hypothalamus. The neurohypophysis stores and releases peptide hormones produced in the hypothalamus namely OXYTOCIN and VASOPRESSIN. The adenohypophysis secretes GROWTH HORMONE, GONADOTROPHIN, prolactin (involved in stimulating lactation), ACTH and THYROID stimulating hormones.

placebo an inactive substance, taken as medication, that nevertheless may help to relieve a condition. The change occurs because the patient expects some treatment (even if nothing need, in reality, be done) and an improvement reflects the expectations of the patient.

New drugs are tested in trials against placebos when the effect of the drug is measured against the placebo response which happens, even when there is no active ingredient in the placebo.

placenta the organ attaching the embryo to the UTERUS. It is a temporary feature comprising maternal and embryonic tissues and it allows oxygen and nutrients to pass from the mother's blood to the embryo's blood. There is, however, no direct contact of blood supplies. The embryo also receives salt, glucose, amino acids, some peptides and antibodies, fats and vitamins. Waste molecules from the embryo are removed by diffusion into the maternal circulation. It also stores GLYCOGEN for conversion to glucose if required and secretes hormones to regulate the pregnancy. It is expelled after birth.

placenta praevia when the placenta is situated in the bottom part of the uterus next to or over the cervix. In the later stages of pregnancy there may be placental separation causing bleeding which will require attention. In the more extreme cases, a Caesarian section will be necessary for delivery.

plague any epidemic disease that results in a high death rate. Specifically the Bubonic plague transmitted to man from infected rats by the rat flea.

plantar descriptive term meaning relating to the sole of the foot.

plasma a light-coloured fluid component of BLOOD and in which the various cells are suspended. It contains inorganic salts with protein and some trace substances. One protein present is FIBRINOGEN.

plastic surgery a branch of surgery that deals with the repair or rebuilding of damaged, deformed or missing parts of the body. *Cosmetic* plastic surgery is merely for the improvement of appearance but most is to repair burns, accident damage or congenital defects.

pleura the SEROUS MEMBRANE that covers the lungs (*visceral*) and the inside of the chest wall (*parietal*). The membranes have a smooth surface which is moistened to allow them to slide over each other.

pleural cavity the small space between the PLEURA which slide over each other when breathing in and out. Should gas or fluid enter the cavity due to infection or injury the space increases and may hinder breathing.

pleurectomy removal, by surgery, of part of the PLEURA to overcome PNEUMOTHORAX or to excise diseased areas.

pleurisy (*or* **pleuritis**) inflammation of the PLEURA resulting in pain from deep breathing, and resulting shortness of breath. There is a typical frictional rub heard through a stethoscope. Pleurisy is often due to pneumonia in the adjacent lung and is always associated with disease in the lung, diaphragm, chest wall or abdomen e.g. tuberculosis, abscesses, bronchial carcinoma etc.

plexus a network formed from intersecting nerves and/or blood vessels, or lymphatic vessels.

pneumoconiosis a general term for a chronic form of lung disease caused by inhaling dust while working. Most of the cases are anthracosis (coal miner's pneumoconiosis), SILICOSIS and asbestosis.

pneumonectomy the surgical removal of a lung performed mainly for cancer but also for tuberculosis.

pneumonia a bacterial infection of the lungs resulting in inflammation and filling of the ALVEOLI with pus and fluid. As a result the lung becomes solid and air cannot enter. The symptoms vary depending upon how much of the lung is unavailable for respiration, but commonly there will be chest pain, coughing, breathlessness, fever and possibly CYANOSIS. Pneumonia may be caused by several bacteria, viruses or fungi, but bacterial infection is commonest. Bronchopneumonia affects the bronchi and bronchioles; lobar pneumonia the whole lobes of the lung(s). Antibiotic treatment is usually effective although it helps to know which is the infecting organism, to provide the most specific treatment. (*See also* VIRAL PNEUMONIA).

pneumonitis inflammation of the lungs by chemical or physical agents.

pneumothorax air in the PLEURAL CAVITY, which enters via a wound in the chest wall or lung. When this happens, the lung collapses but if the air is absorbed from the pleural cavity the lung reinflates.

pock a small eruption on the skin, which may contain pus, typical of chickenpox and smallpox.

poliomyelitis (*or* **infantile paralysis**, **polio**) an infectious disease, caused by a virus, which attacks the central nervous system. The virus is taken in by mouth, passes through the digestive system, is excreted with the faeces and hands may be contaminated, leading to further spread. The incubation period is 7 to 12 days and there are several types of condition, depending upon the severity of the attack. In some cases the symptoms resemble a stomach upset or influenza; in others there is in addition some stiffness of muscles. Paralytic poliomyelitis is less common, resulting in muscle weakness and paralysis while the most serious cases involve breathing when the diaphragm and related muscles are affected (bulbar poliomyelitis). Treatment of the disease involves relief of the symptoms including bed rest, and for the bulbar form, a respirator may be required.

Immunization is highly effective and the disease has almost been eradicated in most countries. However, booster doses are advisable when visiting countries with a high incidence of the disease.

polydactyly the condition in which there are extra fingers or toes.

polydipsia an intense thirst, abnormally so. It is a characteristic symptom of DIABETES MELLITUS and certain other diseases.

polyp a growth from a mucous membrane and attached to it by a stalk. Most are benign but may cause obstructions or infections. They commonly occur in the sinuses, nose, or possibly the bladder or bowels. Their removal is usually straightfor-

ward, unless a more extensive operation proves necessary to reach the affected organ.

polyuria the passing of a larger than normal quantity of urine which is also usually pale in colour. It may be due merely to a large fluid intake, or to a condition such as DIABETES, or a kidney disorder.

pons tissue that joins parts of an organ, e.g. the *pons Varolii,* a part of the brainstem links various parts of the brain including the medulla oblongata and thalamus.

pore a small opening, e.g. sweat pores.

portal vein a vein within the hepatic portal system that carries blood to the liver from other abdominal organs (stomach, spleen, intestine, etc.). It is atypical in that it does not take blood directly to the heart but ends in a capillary network.

possetting the term for the normal habit of some quite healthy babies to regurgitate small amounts of a recently-taken meal.

post mortem *see* AUTOPSY.

postpartum the term meaning relating to the first few days after birth.

poultice (*or* **fomentation**) hot, moist material applied to the body to soften the skin, soothe irritations, ease pain or increase the circulation locally.

pox pus-filled pimples as in chickenpox or smallpox. Also the small pitlike depressions that are scars of smallpox.

precancerous any condition that is not malignant but is known will become so if left untreated.

pre-eclampsia the development of high blood pressure in pregnancy, sometimes with OEDEMA which unless treated may result in ECLAMPSIA.

pregnancy the period of time, lasting approximately 280 days from the first day of the last menstrual period, during which a woman carries a developing foetus. Signs of a pregnancy include cessation of menstruation, increase in size of the breasts, MORNING SICKNESS, and later in the pregnancy the obvious sign of enlargement of the abdomen. A foetal heartbeat and movements also follow later. Many of these changes are hormone-controlled, by progesterone (from the OVARY and PLACENTA).

pregnancy test various tests are used to check for pregnancy, most based on the presence of CHORIONIC GONADOTROPHIN HORMONE in the urine.

premature birth a birth occurring before the end of the normal full term. The definition refers to babies weighing less than 2kg. In many cases the cause is unknown but in some it may be due to PRE-ECLAMPSIA, kidney or heart disease or multiple pregnancy. Premature babies often require incubator care.

premedication drugs given to a patient before an operation in which an anaesthetic is used. It is usually a sedative and a drug to reduce secretions of the lungs which could be inhaled otherwise.

premenstrual tension (or syndrome) the occurrence for up to ten days before menstruation, of such symptoms as headache, nervousness and irritability, emotional disturbance, depression, fatigue with other physical manifestations such as swelling of legs and breasts, and constipation. The condition usually disappears soon after menstruation begins. The cause is not known although the hormone PROGESTERONE is probably involved in some way.

premolar two teeth between the canines and molars on each side of the jaw.

prenatal diagnosis see AMNIOCENTESIS.

prepuce see FORESKIN.

presentation the point, during LABOUR, at which some part of the foetus lies at the mouth of the womb. In the majority of cases the head presents, but see BREECH PRESENTATION.

pressure sores see BED SORES.

prickly heat (**heat rash** or **miliaria**) an itchy rash due to small red spots which are minute vesicles caused by the blocking of sweat or sebaceous glands in the skin. Scratching may produce infection but the condition itself is not serious.

prima gravida the technical term for a woman in her first pregnancy.

progesterone a steroid hormone that is vital in pregnancy. It is produced by the CORPUS LUTEUM of the OVARY when the lining of the uterus is prepared for the implanting of an egg cell. Progesterone is secreted under the control of other hormones (prolactin from the anterior PITUITARY, and luteinizing hormone also from the pituitary which stimulates ovulation and formation of the corpus luteum) until the placenta adopts this role later in the pregnancy. The function of progesterone is to maintain the uterus and ensure no further eggs are produced. Small amounts of this hormone are also produced by the testes.

prognosis a forecast of the likely outcome of a disease, based upon the patient's condition and the course of the disease in other patients at other times.

prolapse a moving down of an organ or tissue from its normal position due to the supporting tissues weakening. This may happen to the lower end of the bowel (in children) or the uterus and vagina in women who have sustained some sort of injury during childbirth. In the latter case prolapse may result in the uterus itself showing on the outside. Surgery can shorten the supporting ligaments and narrow the vaginal opening.

prolapsed intervertebral disc (**slipped disc**) the intervertebral disc provides cushioning for the brain and spinal cord and is composed of an outer fibrous layer over a pulpy centre. A slipped disc is caused by the inner layer being pushed through the fibrous layer to impinge upon nerves, causing pain (commonly lumbago or sciatica). The prolapse usually occurs during sudden twisting or bending of the backbone and is more likely to occur during middle age.

prone lying face downwards.

prophylactic some treatment or action that is taken to avoid disease or a condition, e.g. taking a medication to prevent angina.

prostaglandin (PG) a group of compounds derived from essential fatty acids that act in a way that is similar to hormones. They are found in most body tissues (but especially semen) where they are released as local regulators (in the uterus, brain, lungs, etc.). A number have been identified, two of which act antagonistically on blood vessels. PGE

causing dilation, PGF constriction. Certain prostaglandins cause uterine contraction in labour, and others are involved in the body's defence mechanisms.

prostatectomy surgical excision of the PROSTATE GLAND, performed to relieve urine retention caused by enlargement of the prostate. It is also done to counter poor flow of urine or frequent urination. The operation can be undertaken from several approaches: via the urethra, from the bladder, or from the PERINEUM (for a BIOPSY).

prostate gland a gland in the male reproductive system which is located below the bladder, opening into the URETHRA. Upon ejaculation, it secretes an alkaline fluid into the semen which aids sperm motility. In older men, the gland may become enlarged, causing problems with urination (*see* PROSTATECTOMY).

prostatitis inflammation of the PROSTATE GLAND due to bacterial infection. The symptoms tend to be similar to a urinary infection although in the chronic form obstructions may form necessitating PROSTATECTOMY.

prostheses (*singular* **prosthesis**) artificial devices fitted to the body, ranging from dentures to hearing aids, pacemakers and artificial limbs.

protein a large group of organic compounds containing carbon, hydrogen, oxygen, sulphur and nitrogen, with individual molecules built up of AMINO ACIDS in long POLYPEPTIDE chains. Globular protein includes ENZYMES, ANTIBODIES, carrier proteins (e.g. HAEMOGLOBIN) some HORMONES, etc. Fibrous proteins have elasticity and strength and are found in muscle, connective tissue and also chromosomes.

Proteins are thus vital to the body and are synthesized from their constituent amino acids, which are obtained from digestion of dietary protein.

proteinuria the condition in which protein (usually albumin) is found in the urine. It is important because it may signify heart or kidney disease. Proteinuria may also occur with fever, severe anaemia and intake of certain drugs or poisons.

pruritus another term for itching, of whatever origin.

psoriasis a chronic skin disease for which the cause is unknown and the treatment is palliative. The affected skin appears as itchy, scaly red areas, starting usually around the elbows and knees. It often runs in families and may be associated with anxiety, commencing usually in childhood or adolescence. Treatment involves the use of ointments and creams with some drugs and vitamin A.

psychiatrist a qualified physician who deals with mental disorders including emotional and behavioural problems.

psychiatry the study of mental disorders, their diagnosis, treatment/management and prevention.

psychoanalysis a method of treating mental ill-health by uncovering repressed fears, and dealing with them in the conscious mind. This school of psychology began with Sigmund Freud.

psychogeriatrics the branch of psychiatry dealing with mental ill-health in old people.

psychology the study of the mind, its

working and resulting behaviour patterns. There are many schools of psychology including experimental (laboratory experiments to study topics such as learning), PSYCHOANALYSIS, ethology (study of animal behaviour in the natural environment) and behaviourism.

psychopathic when a person has a mental disorder resulting in antisocial behaviour with little or no guilt for any such acts committed. In addition, psychopaths do not show any ability for showing affection, sympathy or love to others and punishment does not deter a repeat of any criminal act.

psychosis a very serious state of mental ill-health, essentially insanity. The sufferer loses touch with reality and may suffer delusions and hallucinations. Schizophrenia and manic depressive psychosis are two important psychoses.

psychosomatic the term meaning relating to both mind and body and used most often for illnesses and conditions that result from the effects of excessive emotional stress upon the body. Numerous physical ailments can be triggered in this way, from nausea, abdominal pains, ulcer and asthma to dizziness, insomnia and ARRHYTHMIA. The causes of the stress may be even more numerous but essentially fall into categories such as personal/marital; occupational; social. Although psychological treatment may help, attention to the physical symptoms is more effective.

psychotherapy the treatment of mental disorders, or the mental part of an ailment by psychological means, i.e.

by concentrating upon and working through the mind. There are several approaches to this method of treatment including psychoanalysis, group therapy and behavioural therapy.

psychotropic drugs drugs that affect the mind and its moods, e.g. antidepressants, sedatives and stimulants.

puberty the changes that occur in boys and girls around the age of 10 to 14 which signify the beginnings of sexual maturity, and the subsequent functioning of reproductive organs. It is apparent through the appearance of secondary sexual characteristics such as a deepening of the voice in boys and growth of breasts in girls. In addition, girls commence menstruation and in boys the size of testicles increases. In both sexes body shape changes noticeably and body hair grows. The changes are initiated by PITUITARY GLAND hormones acting on the ovaries and testes.

pubis one of three bones, and the most anterior, that makes up each half of the pelvic girdle.

pulmonary relating to the lungs.

pulmonary embolism a condition involving the blocking of the pulmonary artery or a branch of it by an EMBOLUS (usually a blood clot). The clot usually originates from PHLEBOTHROMBOSIS of the leg. The seriousness of the attack relates to the size of the clot. Large pulmonary emboli can be immediately fatal. Smaller ones may cause death of parts of the lung, PLEURISY and coughing up of blood. Anticoagulant drugs are used in minor cases; streptokinase may be used to dissolve the clot or immediate surgery

may be necessary. Several embolisms may produce PULMONARY HYPERTENSION.

pulmonary hypertension an increase in blood pressure in the pulmonary artery due to increased resistance to the flow of blood. The cause is usually disease of the lung (such as BRONCHITIS, EMPHYSEMA, *see also* PULMONARY EMBOLISM) and the result is that the pressure increases in the right ventricle, enlarging it, producing pain with the possibility of heart failure.

pulmonary oedema gathering of fluid in the lungs caused by, for example, MITRAL STENOSIS.

pulmonary stenosis a narrowing of the outlet from the heart to the pulmonary artery via the right ventricle which may be congenital or due, more rarely, to rheumatic fever. Severe cases can produce ANGINA, fainting and enlargement of the heart with eventual heart failure. Surgery is necessary to clear the obstruction.

pulse the regular expansion and contraction of an artery as a fluid wave of blood passes along, originating with the contraction of the heart and blood leaving the left ventricle. It is detected on arteries near the surface, e.g. the radial artery on the wrist and decreases with a reduction in the size of artery so that the capillaries are under a steady pressure (hence the reason why venous flow is also steady).

pupil the circular opening in the IRIS which permits light into the lens in the EYE.

purgative drugs or other treatments taken to evacuate the bowels. These may be grouped by their mode of action, LAXATIVES providing a gentle effect. Purgatives work by increasing the muscular contractions of the intestine or by increasing the fluid in the intestine.

pus the liquid found at an infected site (abscess, ulcer, etc.). It is coloured white, yellow or greenish and consists of dead white blood cells, living and dead bacteria and dead tissue.

pyelitis inflammation of part of the kidney, the pelvis. (This is the area from which urine drains into the ureter). The cause is usually a bacterial infection (commonly *E. coli*) and sometimes occurs as a complication of pregnancy. The symptoms include pain in the loins, high temperature, loss of weight, but it does respond to antibiotics. It is usually the case that the infection is not limited to the pel-

vis but all the kidney hence a more accurate term is *pyelonephritis*.

pyloric stenosis a narrowing of the PYLORUS which limits the movement of food from the stomach to the duodenum, resulting in vomiting. It may be accompanied by distension and peristalsis of the stomach, visible through the abdominal wall. A continuation of the condition causes weight loss, dehydration and ALKALOSIS. It is often due to an ulcer or cancer near the pylorus which requires surgery.

pylorus the lower end of the stomach where food passes into the duodenum and at which there is a ring of muscle, the *pyloric sphincter*.

pyrexia another term for FEVER.

Q

quadriceps the large thigh muscle, which is divided into four distinct parts, and is responsible for movements of the knee joint.

quadriplegia paralysis of all four limbs of the body.

quarantine a period of time in which a person (or animal) who has, or is suspected of having, an infectious disease is isolated from others to prevent the spread of the infection.

Quartan fever the recurrent fever, which usually occurs every fourth day, associated with MALARIA.

quickening the first movements of a

baby in the womb which are perceived by the mother usually around the fourth month of pregnancy.

quinine a colourless alkaloid derived from the bark of certain (cinchona) trees which is a strong antiseptic especially effective against the malarial parasite. It was formerly widely used in the treatment of malaria but has now largely been replaced because it is toxic in larger doses. In small amounts it has a stimulating effect and is used in 'tonic' water.

quinsy the medical name for this condition is *pentonsillar abscess* and it is a complication of TONSILLITIS. A pus-filled abscess occurs near the tonsil, causing great difficulty in swallowing, and this may require surgical lancing.

R

rabies (also known as *hydrophobia*) a very severe and fatal disease affecting the central nervous system which occurs in dogs, wolves, cats and other canine animals. Human beings are infected through the bite of a *rabid* animal, usually a dog. The onset of symptoms varies from ten days to up to a year from the time of being bitten. Characteristically, the person becomes irritable `and depressed, swallowing and breathing difficulties develop, there are periods of great mental excitement, increased salivation and muscular spasms of the throat. Eventually, even the sight of water causes severe muscular spasms, convulsions and paralysis, and death follows within about four days. Treatment consists of thorough cleansing of the bite and injections of rabies vaccine, antiserum and immunoglobulin. As the United Kingdom is currently free of rabies, vigilant quarantine and other regulations involving the movement of animals, are in force.

radiation sickness any illness which is caused by harmful radiation from radioactive substances. This may be a complication of radiotherapy for cancer and produces symptoms of nausea, vomiting and sometimes itchiness of the skin. Antihistamine drugs and tranquillizers such as chlorpromazine are used to alleviate the condition.

radical treatment treatment aimed at the complete cure of a condition (i.e. 'to the root'), rather than the alleviation of symptoms. In contrast, *conservative treatment* is directed towards the minimum interference necessary to keep a condition under control.

radiograph an image produced by x-rays on a film. *Radiography* is the diagnostic technique used to examine the body using X-rays.

radiologist a doctor specialized in the interpretation of X-rays and other diagnostic records.

radiology the branch of medicine concerned with the use of X-rays.

radiotherapy the therapeutic use of penetrating radiation including X-rays, beta rays and gamma rays. These may be derived from X-ray machines or radioactive isotopes and are especially employed in the treatment of cancer. The main disadvantages of radiotherapy is that there may be damage to normal, healthy surrounding tissues.

radium a radioactive metallic element which occurs naturally and emits alpha, beta and gamma rays as it decays. The gamma rays derived from radium are used in the treatment of cancer.

radius the shorter outer bone of the forearm the other being the *ulna*

rash an eruption of the skin which is usually short-lived and consists of reddened, perhaps itchy area or raised red spots.

radon a radioactive gas produced when RADIUM decays. *Radon seeds* are small, sealed capsules which are used in radiotherapy for cancer.

rat bite fever two types of infectious disease which are contracted following the bite of a rat. The first type is caused by either of two kinds of bacteria and produces symptoms of fever, skin rash and joint and muscle pains. The second type is caused by a fungus and produces similar symptoms and vomiting. Both diseases are treated with penicillin.

recessive gene a gene whose character will only be expressed if paired with a similar gene (allele).

recombinant DNA DNA (deoxyribonucleic acid) containing genes which have been artificially combined by the techniques of GENETIC ENGINEERING. Recombinant DNA technology has become synonymous with genetic engineering.

rectum the final portion of the large intestine between the colon and anal canal in which faeces are stored prior to elimination.

red blood cell *see* ERYTHROCYTE.

referred pain (synalgia) pain felt in another part of the body at a distance from the site at which it might be expected. An example is certain heart conditions which cause pain in the left arm and fingers. The condition arises because some sensory nerves share common routes in the central nervous system hence stimulation of one causes an effect in another.

reflex action an unconscious movement which is brought about by relatively simple nervous circuits in the central nervous system. In its simplest form it involves a single *reflex arc* of one receptor and sensory nerve which forms a *synapse* in the BRAIN or SPINAL cord with a motor nerve which then transmits the impulse to a muscle or gland to bring about a response. However some reflex actions are more complicated than this, involving several neurones. Examples are the *plantar reflex* of the toes, when the sole of the foot is stroked, the *knee jerk reflex* and the reflex pupil of the eye which contracts suddenly when a light is directed upon its surface. The presence or absence of reflexes give an indication of the condition of the nervous system and are pointers to the presence or absence of disease or damage.

refractory a condition which does not respond to treatment.

refractory period the time taken for a nerve or muscle cell to recover after an electrical impulse has passed along, or following contraction. During this time, the nerve or muscle cell is unable to respond to a further stimulus.

regression in psychiatry, this refers to a reversion to a more immature form of behaviour. In medicine the term refers to the stage in the course of a disease when symptoms cease and the patient recovers.

regurgitation the bringing up of swallowed undigested food from the stomach to the mouth (*see also* POSSETTING).

The term is also used to describe the backward flow of blood in the heart if one or more valves is diseased and defective.

Reiter's syndrome a disease of unknown cause, affecting men, which produces symptoms of URETHRITIS, CONJUNCTIVITIS and ARTHRITIS. It may also produce other symptoms including fever and diarrhoea and it is suspected that the cause may be a virus.

rejection this is a term used in transplant medicine describing the situation in which the immune system of the recipient individual rejects and destroys an organ or tissue grafted from a donor. Various drugs, e.g. *cyclosporin A*, are given to the recipient to dampen down the immune system and reduce the risk of rejection.

relapse the return of the symptoms of a disease from which a person had apparently recovered or was in the process of recovery.

relapsing fever a disease caused by spirochaete bacteria of the genus *Borrelia* which is transmitted to man by lice and ticks. The disease is characterized by recurrent bouts of fever accompanied by headache, joint and muscle pains and nosebleeds. The first attack lasts for about two to eight days and further milder bouts occur after 3 to ten days. Treatment is by means of bed rest and with erythromycin and tetracycline drugs.

remission a period during the course of a disease when symptoms have lessened or disappeared.

REM sleep this stands for *R*apid *E*ye

*M*ovement SLEEP and describes a phase when the eyeballs move rapidly behind closed eyelids. This appears to be the phase during which dreaming occurs.

renal describing or relating to the kidneys.

repetitive strain injury *see* TENDINITIS.

reproductive system the name given to all the organs involved in reproduction. In males these comprise the testes, vasa deferentia, prostate gland, seminal vesicles, urethra and penis. In females, the reproductive system consists of the ovaries, Fallopian tubes, womb (uterus), vagina and vulva (*see individual entries*).

resection a surgical operation in which part of an organ, or any body part, is removed.

resistance the degree of natural immunity which an individual possesses against a certain disease or diseases. The term is also applied to the degree with which a disease or disease-causing organism can withstand treatment with drugs such as a course of antibiotics.

resonance the quality and increase of sound produced by striking the body over an air-filled structure. If resonance is decreased compared to normal this is termed *dullness* and if increased *hyper-resonance*. Tapping the body, often the chest, to determine the degree of resonance, is called *percussion*.

respiration the whole process by which air is drawn into and out of the lungs during which oxygen is absorbed into the bloodstream and carbon dioxide and water are given off. *External respiration* is the actual process of breathing and the exchange of gases which takes place in the lungs. *Internal respiration* is the process by which oxygen is given up from the blood circulation to the tissues, in all parts of the body, and carbon dioxide is taken up to be transported back to the lungs and eliminated.

The process of drawing air into the lungs is known as *inhalation* or *inspiration* and expelling it out as *exhalation* or *expiration*. The rate at which this occurs is known as the *respiratory rate* and it is about 18 times a minute in a static healthy adult.

respirator one of a number of different devices used to assist or take over RESPIRATION, especially when the muscles which should normally be involved are paralysed, as in some forms of POLIOMYELITIS.

respiratory distress syndrome this usually refers to a condition arising in newborn babies, especially those which are premature, being particularly common in infants born between 32-37 weeks gestation. It is also known as *hyaline membrane disease* and is characterized by rapid shallow laboured breathing. It arises because the lungs are not properly expanded and lack a substance (known as surfactant) necessary to bring their expansion about.

Adults may suffer from *adult respiratory distress syndrome* in which there is PULMONARY OEDEMA and a high mortality rate.

respiratory syncitial virus generally called RS Virus, this is the main cause of BRONCHIOLITIS and pneumonia in babies under the age of 6 months

respiratory system all the organs and tissues involved in RESPIRATION including the nose, pharynx, larynx, trachea, bronchi, bronchioles, lungs and diaphragm, along with the muscles which bring about respiratory movements (*see individual entries*).

resuscitation reviving a person in whom heart beat and breathing has ceased. See ARTIFICIAL RESPIRATION and CARDIAC MASSAGE.

retardation the slowing down of an activity or a process, often referring to mental subnormality or 'backwardness'.

retina the layer which lines the interior of the eye. The retina itself consists of two layers the inner one next to the cavity of the eyeball containing the light-sensitive cells, the RODS and CONES, and also nerve fibres. This layer receives light directed onto its surface by the lens. The outer layer of the retina next to the *choroid* contains pigmented cells which prevent the passage of light (*See also* EYE).

retinol *see* VITAMIN A.

retractor one of a number of different surgical instruments designed to pull apart the cut edges of an incision to allow greater operating access.

retroflexion the bending backwards of a part of an organ, particularly the upper portion of the uterus (*compare* RETROVERSION).

retroversion an abnormal position of the uterus in which the whole organ is tilted backwards instead of forwards, as is normally the case. A *retroverted uterus* occurs in about 20% of women (*see* RETROFLEXION).

retrovirus a type of virus containing RNA (ribonucleic acid) which is able to introduce its genetic material into the DNA of body cells. These viruses are suspected causal agents in the development of certain cancers.

Reye's syndrome a rare disorder, of unknown cause, which affects children and seems to follow on from a viral infection such as chickenpox, often manifesting itself during the recovery phase. The symptoms include vomiting, high fever, delirium, convulsions leading to coma and death, the mortality rate being about 25%. Among those who survive, about half suffer some brain damage. It has been suggested that aspirin may be implicated in the development of this condition and this drug is not now recommended for children under the age of 12.

Rhesus factor *see* BLOOD GROUP.

rheumatic fever a severe disease affecting children and young adults which is a complication of upper respiratory tract infection with bacteria known as *Haemolytic streptococci*. The symptoms include fever, joint pain and ARTHRITIS which progresses from joint to joint, a characteristic red rash known as *Erythema marginatum* and also painless nodules which develop beneath the skin over bony protuberances such as the elbow, knee and back of the wrist. In addition there is CHOREA and inflammation of the heart including the muscle, valves and membranes. The condition may lead to rheumatic heart disease in which there is scarring and inflammation of heart structures. There is sometimes a need for heart valves to be replaced in later life.

rheumatism a general term used to describe aches and pains in joints and muscles.

rheumatoid arthritis the second most common form of joint disease after OSTEOARTHRITIS which usually affects the feet, ankles, fingers and wrists. The condition is diagnosed by means of X-rays which show a typical pattern of changes around the inflamed joints known as *rheumatoid erosions*. At first there is swelling of the joint and inflammation of the SYNOVIAL MEMBRANE (the membraneous sac which surrounds the joint), followed by erosion and loss of cartilage and bone. In addition, a blood test reveals the presence of *serum rheumatoid factor antibody* which is characteristic of this condition. The condition varies greatly in its degree of severity but at its worst can be progressive and seriously disabling. In other people, after an initial active phase, there may be a long period of remission.

rheumatology the branch of medicine concerned with diseases of the joints and associated tissues and structures. The medical specialist in this field is known as a *rheumatologist*.

rhinitis inflammation of the mucous membrane of the nose such as occurs with colds and allergic reactions.

rhinoplasty any one of a large number of RNA - containing viruses which cause upper respiratory tract infections including the common cold.

ribs 12 pairs of thin, slightly twisted and curved bones which form the thoracic rib cage which protects the lungs and heart. The *true ribs* are the first seven pairs which are each connected to the STERNUM at the front by a costal CARTILAGE. The *false ribs* are the next three pairs are indirectly connected to the sternum as each is attached by its cartilage to the rib above. The *floating ribs* are the last two pairs which are unattached and end freely in the muscle of the thoracic wall. At the backbone, the head of each rib articulates with one of the 12 thoracic vertebrae.

rickets this is a disease affecting children which involves a deficiency of VITAMIN D. Vitamin D can be manufactured in the skin in the presence of sunlight but dietary sources are important especially where sunlight is lacking. The disease is characterized by soft bones which bend out of shape and cause deformities.

Bones are hardened by the deposition of calcium salts and this cannot happen in the absence of vitamin D. Treatment consists of giving vitamin D, usually in the form of calciferol, and ensuring that there is an adequate amount in the child's future diet. Vitamin D deficiency in adults causes the condition called OSTEOMALACIA.

rickettsiae a group of microorganisms, which share characteristics in common with both bacteria and viruses and are parasites which occur in lice, fleas and ticks and other arthropods. They can be passed to man by the bites of these animals and are the cause of several serious diseases including TYPHUS, *Rocky Mountain spotted fever* and Q fever.

rigidity especially used to describe stiffness in a limb which is being moved passively, which is a symptom of Parkinson's disease (*see* PARKINSONISM).

rigor a sudden bout of shivering and feeling of coldness which often accompanies the start of a fever.

rigor mortis the stiffening of the body that occurs within eight hours of death due to chemical changes in the muscles.

Ringer's solution a physiological solution containing sodium chloride (salt), potassium chloride and calcium chloride and some other minerals, in the same proportions as in blood serum. It is injected intravenously in people suffering from dehydration and is used to bathe and maintain organs which have been removed for transplant operations.

ringworm this is an infection caused by various species of fungi and is known medically as Tinea. It is classified according to the area affected e.g. *Tinea capitis* which is ringworm of the scalp. Other areas affected are the beard, groin, (dhobie itch), nails and feet (athletes foot).

The infection is typically slightly raised, itchy and with a ring-like appearance. It is highly contagious and the commonest form is athletes foot which usually begins between the toes. The antibiotic drug griseofulvin, taken by mouth, is the normal treatment for ringworm and also antifungal creams applied to the affected areas.

Rinne's test a hearing test that uses a vibrating tuning fork which helps to determine whether deafness is perceptive (nervous) or *conductive* (indicating an obstruction within the ear).

RNA ribonucleic acid which is a complex nucleic acid present mainly in the CYTOPLASM of cells but also in the NUCLEUS. It is involved in the production of proteins and exists in three forms, ribosomal (r), transfer (t) and messenger (m) RNA. In some viruses it forms the genetic material (*see also* DNA).

rod one of the two types of light sensitive cell present in the RETINA of the EYE. The rods enable vision in dim light due to a pigment called *rhodopsin (visual purple)*. This pigment degenerates or bleaches when light is present and regenerates during darkness. In bright light all the pigment bleaches and the rods cannot function. Bleaching of the pigment gives rise to nerve impulses which are sent to the brain and interpreted.

rodent ulcer a slow-growing malignant ulcer which occurs on the face in elderly people usually near the lips, nostrils or eyelids. Skin and underlying tissues and bone are destroyed if the ulcer is untreated. Normally, treatment is by means of surgery and possibly radiotherapy.

rosacea a disease of the skin of the face characterized by a red, flushed appearance and enlargement of the SEBACEOUS GLANDS in the skin. The nose may also enlarge and look red and lumpy (rhinophyma). The cause is unknown but may be aggravated by certain foods or drinks such as an excess of alcohol. Treatment is by means of *tetracycline drugs*.

roseola any rose-coloured rash such as accompanies various infectious diseases e.g. measles.

Rose-waaler rest a diagnostic blood test which is used to detect RHEUMATOID ARTHRITIS.

rotavirus one of a number of viruses which commonly cause gastroenteritis and diarrhoea in young children under the age of 6 years. They infect the lining cells of the SMALL INTESTINE.

rubella *see* GERMAN MEASLES.

rupture the bursting open of an organ, tissue or structure, e.g. ruptured APPENDIX. Also, a popular name for a HERNIA.

S

Sabin vaccine an oral vaccine for POLIOMYELITIS. The appropriate virus is cultured but rendered nonviolent while retaining its ability to stimulate production of antibodies.

sac a structure resembling a bag, e.g. the lungs.

sacral nerves nerves that serve the legs, anal and genital region and which originate from the sacral area of the spinal column. There are five pairs of sacral nerves.

sacral vertebrae the five vertebrae that are fused together form the SACRUM.

sacrum the lower part of the spinal column comprising five fused vertebrae (SACRAL VERTEBRAE) in a triangular shape. The sacrum forms the back wall of the pelvis and articulates with the coccyx below, lumbar vertebrae above and the hips to the sides.

safe period the days in a woman's MENSTRUAL CYCLE when conception is least likely. OVULATION usually occurs midway through the cycle, about 15 days before onset of menstruation, and the fertile period is about 5 days before and 5 after ovulation. Providing periods are regular, it can be calculated when intercourse is unlikely to result in PREGNANCY.

saliva an alkaline liquid present in the mouth to keep the mouth moist, aid swallowing of food and through the presence of amylase enzymes (ptyalin) to digest starch. It is secreted by the SALIVARY GLANDS and in addition to ptyalin, contains water, mucus and buffers (to minimise changes in acidity).

salivary glands three pairs of glands; parotid, submandibular and sublingual, that produce saliva. The stimulus to produce saliva can be the taste, smell, sight or even thought of food.

Salk vaccine a vaccine against POLIOMYELITIS administered by injection. The virus is treated with formalin which renders it unable to cause the disease but it still prompts the production of antibodies.

Salmonella infections FOOD POISONING due to *Salmonella*, a genus of Gram-negative (*see* GRAM'S STAIN) rodlike bacteria.

salpingectomy the surgical excision of a FALLOPIAN TUBE. The removal of both produces sterilization.

salpingitis inflammation of a tube, usually the Fallopian tube by bacterial infection. It may originate in the vagina or uterus, or be carried in the

blood. Peritonitis can ensue. Severe cases may cause a blockage of the Fallopian tubes resulting in sterility.

salpingostomy the clearing of a blocked FALLOPIAN TUBE, which the blocked part is removed surgically.

sanguineous containing blood, covered or stained with blood.

sarcoma *see* CANCER.

scab a crust that forms over an injury (scratch, sore etc.) during the body's healing processes. The scab consists of FIBRIN, dried blood, SERUM or pus and epithelial cells. Healing occurs beneath the protective scab which falls of when the process is complete. Scabs due to infections occur e.g. on the face, with no previous sign.

scabies a skin infection causing severe itching. It is due to the mite *Sarcoptes scabiei* which burrows into the skin, lays eggs, and the resulting larvae cause the itching. The areas of the body affected are the skin between fingers, wrists, buttocks and genitals.

scalds *see* BURNS.

scan examination of the body using one of a number of techniques, such as COMPUTERIZED TOMOGRAPHY AND ultrasonography (*see* ULTRASOUND).

scaphoid bone a bone of the wrist outside the thumb side of the hand.

scapula the shoulder blade. A triangular bone and one of a pair forming the shoulder girdle.

scar a mark left after a wound heals due to tissues not repairing completely, and being replaced by a fibrous connective tissue.

scarlet fever an infectious disease, mainly of childhood, caused by the bacterium *Streptococcus*. Symptoms show after a few days and include sickness, sore throat, fever and a scarlet rash that may be widespread. Antibiotics are effective and also prevent any complications e.g. inflammation of the kidneys.

schistosomiasis (*or* **bilharziasis**) a parasitic infection caused by blood flukes (*Schistosoma*). Man is infected with the larvae of the fluke that enter through the skin from infected water. The adult then settle in blood vessels of the intestine or bladder. Subsequent release of eggs causes anaemia, diarrhoea, dysentery, enlargement of the spleen and liver and cirrhosis of the liver.

The disease can be treated with drugs but preventative measures are preferable. Schistosomiasis affects millions worldwide, particularly in the Far and Middle East, South America and Africa.

schizophrenia any one of a large group of severe mental disorders typified by gross distortion of reality, disturbance in language and breakdown of thought processes, perceptions and emotions. Delusions and hallucinations are usual, as are apathy, confusion, incontinence and strange behaviour. No single cause is known but genetic factors are probably important. Drug therapy has improved the outlook markedly over recent years.

sciatica pain in the sciatic nerve, and therefore felt in the back of the thigh, leg and foot. The commonest cause is a PROLAPSED INTERVERTEBRAL DISC pressing on a nerve root, but it may also be due to ankylosing SPONDYLITIS and other conditions.

sclera the outer layer of the eyeballs which is white and fibrous same at the front of the eye when it becomes the transparent CORNEA.

scleritis inflammation of the white of the eye (SCLERA).

scleroderma a condition in which connective tissue hardens and contracts. The tissue may be the skin, heart, kidney, lung etc. and the condition may be localized or it may spread throughout the body, eventually being fatal. If the skin is affected, it becomes tough and patchily pigmented and may lead to stiff joints and wasting muscles.

sclerosis hardening of tissue, usually after inflammation leading to parts of organs being hard and of no use. It is applied commonly to such changes in the nervous system (MULTIPLE SCLEROSIS); in other organs it is termed FIBROSIS or CIRRHOSIS

sclerotherapy a treatment for VARICOSE VEINS. An irritant solution is injected, causing FIBROSIS of the vein lining and its eventual removal by THROMBOSIS and scarring.

screening test a programme of tests carried out on a large number of apparently healthy people to find those who may have a particular disease, e.g. cervical smears to detect the precancerous stage of cervical cancer.

scrofula TUBERCULOSIS of the LYMPH NODES in the neck which form sores and scars after healing. It is now an uncommon condition, but drug treatment is effective.

scrotum the sac that contains the testicles and holds them outside the body, to permit production and storage of sperm at a temperature lower than that of the abdomen.

scrum-pox a bacterial (IMPETIGO) or viral (HERPES SIMPLEX) infection of the face, common to rugby players occurring probably through facial contact in the scrum or communal changing facilities.

scurvy a deficiency disease caused by a lack of VITAMIN C (ascorbic acid) due to a dietary lack of fruit and vegetables. Symptoms begin with swollen, bleeding gums and then subcutaneous bleeding, bleeding into joints, ulcers, anaemia and then fainting, diarrhoea and trouble with major organs. Untreated, it is fatal, but nowadays it is easily prevented, or cured should it arise, through correct diet or administration of the vitamin.

sebaceous cyst a cyst formed in the duct of a SEBACEOUS GLAND of the skin.

sebaceous gland any of the minute glands in the skin that secrete an oily substance called SEBUM. The glands open into hair follicles. Activity of the glands varies with age, puberty being the most active period.

seborrhoea excessive production of SEBUM by the SEBACEOUS GLANDS producing either a build up of dry scurf or oily deposits on the skin. The condition often leads to the development of ACNE.

sebum the secretion formed by the SEBACEOUS GLANDS, which forms a thin oily film on the skin, preventing excessive dryness. It also has an antibacterial action.

secondary sexual characteristics the physical features that develop at puberty. In girls, the breasts and genitals increase in size and pubic hair grows. Boys grow pubic hair and facial hair, the voice breaks and the genitals become adult size.

secretin a polyPEPTIDE hormone pro-

duced by the lining of the DUODENUM and JEJUNUM in response to acid from the stomach. It stimulates production of alkaline pancreatic juice, and BILE secretion by the liver.

section cutting in surgery, e.g. an abdominal section.

Also a thin slice of a specimen as used in microscopy.

sedative a drug that lessens tension and anxiety. Sedatives are hypnotic drugs, e.g. barbiturates, given in doses lower than would bring on sleep. They may be used to combat pain, sleeplessness, spasms, etc.

semen the fluid that contains the sperm which is ejaculated from the penis during copulation.

senile dementia an organic mental disorder of the elderly involving generalized atrophy of the brain. The result is a gradual deterioration with loss of memory, impaired judgement, confusion, emotional outbursts and irritability. The degree of the condition may vary considerably.

sensation a feeling. The result of stimulation of a sensory receptor producing a nerve impulse which travels on an afferent fibre to the brain.

sensitivity with reference to a SCREENING TEST, the proportion of people with the disease who are identified by the test.

sensitization a change in the body's response to foreign substances. With the development of an allergy, a person becomes sensitized to a certain ALLERGEN and then becomes hypersensitive. Similarly it may be an acquired reaction when ANTIBODIES develop in response to an ANTIGEN.

sepsis the destruction of tissues through putrefaction by bacteria-causing disease, or toxins produced by bacteria.

septal defect a hole in the SEPTUM or partition between the left and right sides of the heart, whether in the atria (*see* ATRIUM) or VENTRICLES. This condition is a CONGENITAL disorder caused by an abnormal development of the foetal heart. Whether the defect is atrial or ventricular, it allows incorrect circulation of the blood from left to right, from higher pressure to lower. This is called a *shunt*, and results in too much blood flowing through the lungs. PULMONARY HYPERTENSION results and a large shunt may cause heart failure.

septic affected with SEPSIS.

septicaemia a term used loosely for any type of blood poisoning. Also a systemic infection with PATHOGENS from an infected part of the body circulating in the bloodstream.

septic shock a form of shock that occurs due to SEPTICAEMIA. The toxins cause a drastic fall in blood pressure due to tissue damage and blood clotting. Kidneys, heart and lungs are affected and related symptoms include fever, TACHYCARDIA or even coma. The condition occurs most in those who already have a serious disease such as cancer, DIABETES, or CIRRHOSIS. Urgent treatment is vital, with antibiotics, oxygen and fluids given intravenously.

septum a planar dividing feature within a structure of the body; a partition.

serositis inflammation of a SEROUS MEMBRANE.

serous membrane a membrane lining a large cavity in the body. The membranes are smooth and transparent and the surfaces are moistened by fluid derived from blood or lymph serum (hence the name). Examples are the PERITONEUM and the PERICARDIUM. Each consists of two layers, the *visceral* which surrounds the organs and the *parietal* which lines the cavity. The two portions are continuous and the surfaces are close together, separated by fluid which permits free movement of the organs.

serum a serous fluid. More specifically the clear, sticky fluid that separates from blood and lymph when clotting occurs. In addition to water, serum contains albumin and GLOBULIN with salts, fat, sugar, UREA and other compounds important in disease prevention.

Also, a VACCINE prepared from the serum of a hyperimmune donor for use in protection against a particular infection.

serum sickness a hypersensitive reaction that occasionally occurs several days after injection of foreign SERUM, producing rashes, joint pains, fever and swelling of the lymph nodes. It is due to circulating antigen material to which the body responds. It is not a serious condition.

sessile in description of a tumour or growth, one having no stalk.

sex chromosomes CHROMOSOMES that play a major role in determining the sex of the bearer. Sex chromosomes contain GENES that control the characteristics of the individual, e.g. testes in males, ovaries in females. Women have two X chromosomes while men have one X and one Y chromosomes (*see individual entries*).

sex hormones steroid hormones responsible for the control of sexual development (primary and SECOND-ARY SEXUAL CHARACTERISTICS) and re-productive function. The ovaries and testes are the organs primarily in-volved in hormone production, of which there are three main types: AN-DROGENS, the male sex hormones; OESTROGENS and PROGESTERONE, the female sex hormones.

sex-linked disorders conditions pro-duced because the genes controlling certain characteristics are carried on the SEX CHROMOSOMES, usually the X chromosome. Some result from an abnormal number of chromosomes, e.g. KLINEFELTER'S SYNDROME affect-ing only men, and TURNER'S SYN-DROME affecting only women.

Other disorders such as HAEMO-PHILIA are carried on the X chromo-some and these manifest themselves in men because although the genes are recessive, there is no other X chromosome to mask the recessive type, as is the case with women.

sexually-transmitted diseases *see* VENEREAL DISEASES.

shingles the common name for herpes zoster (*see* HERPES).

shock acute circulatory failure, when the arterial blood pressure is too low to provide the normal blood supply to the body. The signs are a cold, clammy skin, pallor, CYANOSIS, weak rapid pulse, irregular breathing and dilated pupils. There may also be a reduced flow of urine and confusion or lethargy. There are numerous causes of shock from a reduction in blood volume as after burns, exter-nal bleeding, dehydration etc. to re-duced heart activity as in CORONARY THROMBOSIS, PULMONARY EMBOLISM, etc.

Certain other circumstances may produce shock, including severe al-lergic reactions (anaphylactic shock, *see* ANAPHYLAXIS), drugs overdose, emotional shock and so on.

short sight *see* MYOPIA.

shoulder the joint formed by the shoulder blade (SCAPULA) and the up-per end of the humerus. It is a ball-and-socket joint surrounded by a fi-brous capsule strengthened with bands of ligament. The strength of the joint is derived from the associ-ated muscles.

shoulder blade *see* SCAPULA.

shoulder girdle *see* PECTORAL GIRDLE.

Siamese twins also termed conjoined twins; when twins are joined to-gether physically at birth. The condi-tion varies from superficial joining, e.g. by the umbilical vessels, to ma-jor fusion of head, torso and internal organs. The latter cases are inevitably very much more difficult to separate. The condition is caused by foetuses developing from the same OVUM.

sickle cell anaemia a type of inherited, haemolytic ANAEMIA (*see* HAEMOLY-SIS) that is genetically-determined and is the most common hereditary disease in the world. It is caused by a recessive gene and is manifested when this gene is inherited from both parents. One AMINO ACID in the HAEMOGLOBIN molecule is substituted causing the disease which results in an abnormal type of haemoglobin be-ing precipitated in the red blood cells during deprivation of oxygen. This produces the distortion of the cells which are removed from the circula-tion causing anaemia and jaundice.

Many people are carriers due to in-heritance of just one defective GENE and because this confers increased resistance to MALARIA, this gene remains at a high level.

side-effect the additional and unwanted effect(s) of a drug above the intended action. Sometimes side-effects are harmful and may be stronger than anticipated results of the drug, or something quite different.

sigmoid colon the end part of the COLON which is S-shaped.

sigmoidectomy surgical excision of the SIGMOID COLON, performed usually for tumours, diverticular disease (*see* DIVERTICULITIS, DIVERTICULOSIS) or a long and twisted sigmoid colon.

sigmoidoscopy the examination of the SIGMOID COLON and rectum with a special viewing device. The instrument is tubular, with illumination, although modern forms use fibre optics, which are flexible.

silicosis a type of PNEUMOCONIOSIS caused by the inhalation of silica as particles of dust. Silica promotes FIBROSIS of the lung tissue resulting in breathlessness and a greater likelihood to contract tuberculosis. Workers in quarrying, mineral mining, sand blasting, etc. are most susceptible.

sinew the TENDON of a muscle.

sinoatrial node the natural heart PACEMAKER which consists of specialized muscle cells in the right atrium. These cells generate electrical impulses, contract and initiate contractions in the muscles of the heart. The AUTONOMIC NERVOUS SYSTEM supplies the node and certain hormones also have an effect.

sinus in general terms a cavity or channel. Specifically air cavities in bone as in the bones of the face and skull. Also a channel, as in the DURA MATER and which drains venous blood from the brain.

sinusitis inflammation of a SINUS. It usually refers to the sinuses in the face which link with the nose and may therefore be due to a spread of infection from the nose. Headaches and a tenderness over the affected sinus are typical symptoms with a pus-containing discharge from the nose. Persistent infection may necessitate surgery to drain the sinus.

Sjögren's syndrome dryness of the mouth and eyes associated with rheumatoid arthritis. The syndrome is due to the destruction of the salivary glands (and lacrimal glands).

skeleton the rigid, supporting framework of the body that protects organs and tissues, provides muscle attachments, facilitates movement, and produces red blood cells. There are 206 bones divided into the axial skeleton (head and trunk) and the appendicular skeleton (limbs). The types of bone are: long (e.g. humerus), short (e.g. carpals), flat (parts of the cranium) and irregular (e.g. the vertebrae).

skin the outer layer of the body comprising an external EPIDERMIS itself made up of a *stratum corneum* (horny layer) formed of flat cells that rub off, being replaced from below. Beneath this are two more layers (*stratum lucidum* and *stratum granulosum*) which act as intermediate stages between the stratum corneum and a still lower layer, the Malpighian layer.

The Malpighian layer is where the epidermis is produced. The dermis lies beneath the epidermis and then follows subcutaneous tissue composed mainly of fat. The subcutaneous tissue contains glands (sweat, SEBACEOUS, etc.), sensory receptors for pain, pressure and temperature, nerves, muscles and blood capillaries.

skin graft (*see also* GRAFT) a piece of skin taken from another site on the body to cover an injured area, commonly due to burns. The graft is normally taken from elsewhere on the patient's body (*autograft*) but occasionally from someone else (*homograft*). A variety of thicknesses and graft types are used, depending upon the wound.

skull the part of the SKELETON that forms the head and encloses the brain. It is made up of 22 bones, forming the cranium (eight bones) and fourteen in the face and all except the mandible are fused along sutures creating immovable joints. The mandible (lower jaw) articulates close to the ears. A large opening at the base of the skull (FORAMEN magnum) allows the spinal cord to pass from the brain to the trunk of the body.

sleep a state of lower awareness accompanied by reduced metabolic activity and physical relaxation. When falling asleep, there is a change in the brain's electrical activity. This activity can be recorded by an ELECTROENCEPHALOGRAM (EEG). There are high amplitude, low frequency waves (slow-wave sleep) interrupted by short periods of low amplitude, high frequency waves. The periods of high frequency waves are typified by restless sleep with dreams and rapid eye movements, hence the name REM SLEEP, and the EEG is similar to that of a waking person.

REM sleep comprises about 25% of the time asleep.

sleeping sickness (African trypanosomiasis) a parasitic disease found in tropical Africa which is spread through the bite of tsetse flies. The organism responsible is a minute protozoan, *Trypanosoma*, and initially the symptoms consist of a recurring fever, a slight rash, headache and chills. Then follows ANAEMIA, enlarged LYMPH NODES and pain in joints and limbs. Then after some time (possibly years), sleeping sickness itself develops. This is due to the parasites occupying minute blood vessels in the brain resulting in damage, and symptoms of drowsiness and lethargy. Death may follow from weakness or an associated disease.

slipped disc *see* PROLAPSED INTERVERTEBRAL DISC.

slough dead tissue, usually of limited extent, that after infection separates from the healthy tissue of the rest of the body. In cases of GANGRENE it is possible for limbs to be lost.

slow virus one of several viruses that show their effects some time after infection, by which time considerable damage of nerve tissue has occurred, resulting ultimately in death. Some years ago such a virus was found to cause scrapie in sheep and recently bovine spongiform encephalopathy in cows. In man a slow virus is thought to be the cause of CREUTZFELDT-JAKOB DISEASE and a type of MENINGITIS.

small intestine *see* INTESTINE.

smallpox a highly infectious viral disease that has nonetheless been eradicated. Infection results, after about two weeks, in a high fever, head and body aches and vomiting. Eventually red spots appear which change to water and then pus-filled vesicles which on drying out leave scars. The person stays infectious until all scabs are shed. Fever often returns, with DELIRIUM, and although recovery is usual, complications often ensue, e.g. PNEUMONIA. The last naturally-occurring case was in 1977.

smooth muscle *see* INVOLUNTARY MUSCLE.

snow blindness an eye disorder due to excessive exposure to ultraviolet light, e.g. as reflected from a snow field. Covering the eyes for 24 hours is usually an effective treatment.

solar plexus a network of sympathetic nerves and ganglia (*see* GANGLION) behind the stomach, surrounding the coeliac artery. It is a major autonomic PLEXUS of the body where nerves of the sympathetic and parasympathetic nervous system combine (*see individual terms*).

somatic descriptive term meaning relating to the body, as opposed to the mind. More specifically, concerning the *nonreproductive* parts of the body.

somnambulism (sleepwalking) walking and performing other functions during sleep with no recollection upon waking.

sore a common term for an ulcer or an open skin wound.

sound an instrument resembling a rod, with a curved end, that is used to explore a body cavity, e.g. the bladder, or to dilate STRICTURES.

spasm a muscular contraction that is involuntary. Spasms may be part of a more major disorder (e.g. spastic paralysis, convulsions) or they may be specific such as cramp, colic, etc. A heart spasm is known as ANGINA.

spasmolytic a drug that reduces spasms (in SMOOTH MUSCLE) in a number of ways. It may generally depress the CENTRAL NERVOUS SYSTEM, act directly on the muscles in question, or modify the nerve impulses causing the spasm. Spasmolytics are used in the treatment of ANGINA, colic and as BRONCHODILATORS.

spasticity muscular hypertonicity (i.e. an increase in the state of readiness of muscle fibres to contract; an increase in the normal partial contraction) with an increased resistance to stretch. Moderate cases show movement requiring great effort and a lack of normal coordination while slight cases show exaggerated movements that are coordinated.

spastic colon *see* IRRITABLE BOWEL SYNDROME.

spastic paralysis weakness of a limb characterized by involuntary muscular contraction and loss of muscular function. As with SPASTICITY it is due to disease of the nerve fibres that usually control movement and reflexes.

speculum an instrument for use in examination of an opening in the body. The speculum holds open the cavity and may also provide illumination.

speech therapy treatment of patients who are unable to speak coherently. Such patients may have congenital conditions or may have suffered an accident or illness producing a condition requiring therapy.

spermatic the term given to any vessel or structure associated with the testicle.

spermatozoon (*plural* **spermatozoa**) the mature male reproductive cell, or gamete. It has a head with the

HAPLOID nucleus containing half the CHROMOSOME number, and an acrosome (a structure that aids penetration of the egg). Behind the head comes a midpiece with energy-producing MITOCHONDRIA, and then a long tail which propels it forward. A few millilitres of SEMEN is ejaculated during intercourse, containing many millions of spermatozoa.

spermicide a cream, foam, jelly, etc. that kills spermatozoa and which is used in conjunction with a DIAPHRAGM as a contraceptive.

sphenoid bone a bone in the skull that lies behind the eyes.

sphincter a circular muscle around an opening. The opening is closed totally or partially by contraction of the muscle, e.g. the anal sphincter around the anus.

sphygmomanometer the instrument used to measure arterial blood pressure. An inflatable rubber tube is put around the arm and inflated until the blood flow in a large artery stops. This pressure is taken as the SYSTOLIC PRESSURE (i.e. the pressure at each heart beat). The pressure is then released slowly and the point at which the sound heard in the artery changes suddenly is taken as the diastolic pressure (see DIASTOLE).

spina bifida a CONGENITAL malformation in new born babies in which part of the spinal cord is exposed by a gap in the backbone. Many cases are also affected with HYDROCEPHALUS. The symptoms usually include paralysis, incontinence, a high risk of MENINGITIS and mental retardation. There is usually an abnormally high level of ALPHA FETOPROTEIN in the amniotic fluid and since this can be di-

agnosed and then confirmed by AMNIOCENTESIS, it is possible to terminate these pregnancies.

spinal anaesthesia generating anaesthesia by injecting the cerebrospinal fluid around the spinal cord. Of the two types, the epidural (see EPIDURAL ANAESTHESIA) involves injecting into the outer lining of the spinal cord, while *subarachnoid anaesthesia* is produced by injecting between vertebrae in the LUMBAR region of the vertebral column. Spinal anaesthesia is useful for patients who have a condition that precludes a general anaesthetic (e.g. a chest infection or heart disease).

The term is also used for a loss of sensation in a part of the body due to spinal injury.

spinal column (spine, backbone, vertebral column) the bony and slightly flexible column that forms a vital part of the SKELETON. It encloses the SPINAL CORD, articulates with other bones, e.g. the skull and ribs, and provides attachments for muscles.

It consists of bones, the vertebrae, between which are discs of fibrocartilage (the intervertebral discs). From the top, the column comprises 7 cervical, 12 thoracic, 5 lumbar, 5 sacral and 4 coccygeal vertebrae. In adults the last two groups are fused to from the sacrum and coccyx, respectively.

spinal cord the part of the CENTRAL NERVOUS SYSTEM that runs from the brain, through the SPINAL COLUMN. Both GREY and WHITE MATTER are present, the former as an H-shaped core within the latter. A hollow core in the grey matter forms the central canal which contains the cerebrospinal fluid. The cord is covered by ME-

NINGES and it contains both sensory and motor NEURONS. Thirty-one pairs of spinal nerves arise from the cord, passing out between the arches of the vertebrae.

spirometer an instrument used to test how the lungs are working, by recording the volume of air inhaled and exhaled.

spleen a roughly ovoid organ, coloured a deep purple, which is situated on the left of the body, behind and below the stomach. It is surrounded by a peritoneal membrane and contains a mass of lymphoid tissue. MACROPHAGES in the spleen destroy microorganisms by PHAGOCYTOSIS.

The spleen produces lymphocytes, leucocytes, plasma cells and blood platelets (*see individual entries*). It also stores red blood cells for use in emergencies. Release of red blood cells is facilitated by SMOOTH MUSCLE under the control of the SYMPATHETIC NERVOUS SYSTEM, and when this occurs, the familiar pain called *stitch* may be experienced. The spleen removes worn out red blood cells, conserving the iron for further production in the bone marrow. Although the spleen performs many functions, it can be removed without detriment and as a result there is an increase in size of the lymphatic glands.

splenectomy removal of the SPLEEN possibly because of rupture and bleeding.

splenomegaly an abnormal enlargement of the SPLEEN which occurs commonly with blood disorders and parasitic infections.

splint a support that holds a broken bone in the correct and stable posi-

tion until healing is complete.

spondylitis inflammation of the spinal vertebrae - arthritis of the spine. *Ankylosing spondylitis* is a rheumatic disease of the spine and sacroiliac joints (i.e. those of the sacrum and ilium), causing pain and stiffness in the hip and shoulder. It may result in the spine become rigid (*see* KYPHOSIS).

spondylosis degeneration of joints and the intervertebral discs of the spine, producing pain in the neck and LUMBAR region where the joints may actually restrict movement. OSTEOPHYTES are commonly formed and the space occupied by the discs reduced. Physiotherapy may help sufferers, and collars or surgical belts can prevent movement and give support. Surgery may be required occasionally to relieve pressure on nerves, or to fuse joints.

spongiform encephalopathy a neurological disease caused by a SLOW VIRUS and resulting in a spongy degeneration of the brain with progressive dementia. Examples are CREUTZFELDT-JAKOB DISEASE and kuru (a progressive and fatal viral infection seen in New Guinea highland natives which has decreased with the decline in cannibalism).

sprain an injury to ligaments (or muscles, or tendons) around a joint, caused by a sudden overstretching. Pain and swelling may occur and treatment comprises, in the main, avoiding use of the affected joint.

sprue (**psilosis**) essentially a composite deficiency disease due to lack of food being absorbed because of a disease of the intestine, or a metabolic disorder which means fats cannot be absorbed. The symptoms include diarrhoea, inflamed tongue, ANAEMIA and weight loss.

The condition was considered a disease of tropical climates but other versions have been seen. Treatment involves antibiotics, folic acid (to combat the anaemia), vitamins and a high-protein diet. There may be an immediate improvement on returning to a temperate climate.

sputum saliva and mucus from the respiratory tract.

squint (*or* **strabismus**) an abnormal condition in which the eyes are crossed. There are two types, paralytic and non-paralytic. The paralytic type is due to a muscular or neurological malfunction, while a non-paralytic squint is caused by a defect in the actual relative position of the eyes. Some squints can be corrected by surgery.

stagnant loop syndrome when a segment of the SMALL INTESTINE is discontinuous with the rest or when there is an obstruction, either of which causes slow movement through the intestines. The result is bacterial growth with malabsorption and steatorrhoea (passage of fatty stools).

starvation *see* **malnutrition**.

stenosis the abnormal narrowing of a blood vessel, heart valve or similar structure.

stent a device used in surgery to help the healing of two structures that have been joined, by draining away the contents.

sterilization the process of destroying all microorganisms on instruments and other objects by means of heat, radiation, etc.

Also, a surgical operation to render someone incapable of producing children. Men usually undergo a VASECTOMY while in women it can be achieved by cutting and tying the FALLOPIAN TUBES, or removing them. The latter operation is performed via an incision in the abdominal wall or through the vagina.

sternum the breastbone.

steroid one of a group of compounds resembling cholesterol, that are made up of four carbon rings fused together. The group includes the sterols (e.g. cholesterol), BILE acids, some HORMONES, and VITAMIN D. Synthetic versions act like steroid hormones and include derivatives of the glucocorticoids used as anti-inflammatory agents for RHEUMATOID ARTHRITIS; oral contraceptives, usually OESTROGEN and PROGESTERONE derivatives; anabolic steroids such as testosterone used to treat OSTEOPOROSIS and wasting.

stethoscope an instrument used to listen to sounds within the body, particularly the lungs and heart. The simplest type consists of earpieces for the examiner, leading via a tube to a diaphragm placed on the body.

Stevens-Johnson syndrome a common hypersensitivity reaction to SULPHONAMIDE antibiotics, and a form of ERYTHEMA. It produces skin lesions and the eyes and mucosa may ulcerate.

stiffness a condition with numerous causes, that results in a reduced movement in joints and muscles. The cause may be quite straightforward, e.g. physical injury, or it may be due to disease such as RHEUMATISM, MENINGITIS or central nervous system diseases.

stigma a mark or impression upon the skin, possibly one that is typical of a particular disease.

stilboestrol a synthetic OESTROGEN (female sex hormone) with several uses. It relieves menstrual disorders and menopause symptoms. It also proves helpful in treating breast and prostate cancers.

stillbirth the birth of any child that provides no evidence of life.

Still's disease a chronic ARTHRITIS affecting children and causing arthritis in several joints, with fever and a red rash. Some cases develop into ankylosing SPONDYLITIS and there is often muscle wasting. Illness may affect the whole body, complicated by other conditions, e.g. enlargement of the SPLEEN, and PERICARDITIS.

stimulant any drug or other agent that increases the rate of activity of an organ or system within the body. This assumes that the target organ is capable of increased activity which merely requires the necessary stimulus.

stoma (*plural* **stomata**) an opening made in the abdominal surface to accommodate a tube from the colon or ileum. This operation is undertaken because of malignancy or inflammatory bowel diseases, e.g. Crohn's disease.

stomach an expansion of the alimentary canal that lies between the OESOPHAGUS and the DUODENUM. It has thick walls of SMOOTH MUSCLE that contract to manipulate the food, and its exits are controlled by SPHINCTERS, the cardiac anteriorly and the pyloric at the junction with the duodenum (*see* PYLORUS). Mucosal cells in the lining secrete GASTRIC JUICE. The food is reduced to an acidic semi-liquid which is moved on to the duodenum.

The stomach varies in size but its greatest length is roughly 12 inches

and the breadth 4 or 5 inches. Its capacity is approximately 1 to 1 1/2 litres.

stools *see* FAECES.

strangulation the constriction or closure of a passage or vessel. This may be due to the intestine twisting (VOLVULUS), or herniation of the intestine. Strangulation of a blood vessel and/or airway affects the organs being supplied and if vital organs are affected, can prove fatal.

strangury the desire to pass water, which can only be done in a few drops and with accompanying pain. It is symptomatic of an irritation of the base of the bladder by a stone, cancer at this site, or CYSTITIS or PROSTATITIS.

strapping the application of layers of adhesive plaster to cover part of the body and maintain moderate pressure, so as to prevent too much movement and provide rest, as with fractured ribs.

Streptococcus a genus of Gram-positive (*see* GRAM'S STAIN) spherical bacteria that form chains. Many species are responsible for a variety of infections including scarlet fever, ENDOCARDITIS and pneumonia.

stress fracture a FRACTURE created by making excessive demands on the body, as in sport. Treatment involves rest and analgesics for the pain.

stricture a narrowing of a passage in the body, e.g. the URETHRA, OESOPHAGUS, or URETER. It may result from inflammation, a spasm, growth of a tumour or pressure from surrounding organs. In many cases it is due to ulceration and contraction of the subsequent scar tissue. With a urethral stricture, it becomes increasingly difficult to pass urine.

stridor the noise created on breathing in when there is a narrowing of the upper airway, especially the LARYNX.

stroke (*or* **apoplexy**) the physical effects, involving some form of paralysis, that result from an interruption to the brain's blood supply. The effect in the brain is secondary and the cause lies in the heart or blood vessels and may be a THROMBOSIS, EMBOLUS, or HAEMORRHAGE. The severity of a stroke varies greatly from a temporary weakness in a limb, or tingling, to paralysis, coma and death.

St Vitus' dance the former name for Sydenham's CHOREA.

stye a bacterial infection and inflammation of a gland at the base of an eyelash, resulting in a pus-filled cyst.

subarachnoid haemorrhage bleeding into the SUBARACHNOID SPACE due often to a ruptured cerebral ANEURYSM. Initial symptoms are a severe headache, stiff neck, followed by vomiting, drowsiness and there may be a brief period of unconsciousness after the event. Brain damage is possible but severe haemorrhages may result in death.

subarachnoid space the space between the arachnoid and pia mater MENINGES covering the brain and spinal cord. It contains cerebrospinal fluid and blood vessels.

subcutaneous general term meaning beneath the skin.

subdural term meaning below the dura mater, and referring to the space between this and the arachnoid MENINGES around the brain.

subphrenic abscess an abscess occurring beneath the diaphragm and commonly on the right side. It may be due to infection after an operation or perforation of an organ, e.g. a peptic ulcer. Surgery is usually necessary although antibiotics may be effective.

Sudden Infant Death Syndrome (*or* **Cot Death**) the sudden death of a baby, often occurring overnight, from unknown causes. A significant proportion (c. 20% in U.K.) of infant deaths occur this way. Although the cause is unknown numerous suggestions have been put forward from viral infection and allergic reaction to poor breathing control that be particularly susceptible to mild infections. Research continues.

sulphonamide one of a group of drugs containing the chemical group $-SO_2NH_2$. These drugs do not kill bacteria, but prevent bacterial growth and are thus very useful in controlling infections. Some side effects may occur but in general these are outweighed by the benefits.

sunburn skin damage caused by exposure to the ultraviolet rays in sunlight. This may vary from a reddening of the skin and itching to formation of blisters which can cause shock if a large area is affected. Fairskinned people are more susceptible than others and it is advisable to take sun in gradual stages.

sunstroke *see* HEATSTROKE.

supine the position in which someone is lying on their back, face upwards.

suppository medication prepared in a form which enables it to be inserted into the rectum (or vagina). It may be a lubricant, drugs for treatment in the area of the rectum or anus, or for absorption. The suppository has to be inserted beyond the sphincter muscle to ensure retention.

suppuration pus formation, whether on the surface (ulceration) or more deep seated (as with an ABSCESS).

surgeon a qualified practitioner specializing in surgery.

surgery the branch of medicine that through operation treats disease and injuries or deformities.

susceptibility when there is a lack of resistance to disease, due either to poor general health, or a deficiency in defence mechanism because of another condition, e.g. AIDS. Susceptibility can be decreased by vaccination, etc.

suture the means whereby a wound or incision is closed in surgery, using threads of silk or catgut. There are several types of suture to deal with diverse situations.

Also, a type of joint across which there is no movement, e.g. as in the skull, where there are several sutures.

swab a general term applied to a pad of material used in various ways. It can be used to clean wounds, apply medication, remove blood during operations, and obtain samples from infected areas, e.g. throat, for further examination.

sweat see PERSPIRATION.

sweat glands the glands in the EPIDERMIS of SKIN that project into the dermis and are under the control of the sympathetic nervous system (see also PERSPIRATION). The glands occur over most of the body but are especially abundant on the forehead, palms of the hands and soles of the feet and under the arms.

sympathetic the term for a symptom or disease that occurs as a result of disease elsewhere in the body, e.g. injury of one eye and a related inflammation in the other due to them being connected by the lymphatics.

sympathetic nervous system with the parasympathetic nervous system (and acting in opposition to it), this makes up the AUTONOMIC NERVOUS SYSTEM. NORADRENALINE and ADRENALINE are the main NEUROTRANSMITTERS released by its nerve endings. Its functions include raising the heart beat rate, constricting blood vessels and inhibiting secretion of saliva.

symptom any evidence of a disease or disorder.

synapse the junction between two nerve cells, at which there is a minute gap. A nerve impulse bridges the gap via a NEUROTRANSMITTER (see also ACETYLCHOLINE). The chemical diffuses across the gap that connects the axon of one nerve cell to the dendrites of the next. Some brain cells have many thousand synapses.

syncope (fainting) a temporary loss of consciousness due to a fall in blood pressure and reduced supply of blood to the brain. It may occur after standing for a long time (particularly in hot weather), after shock or injury. Typical signs before an attack are sweating and light-headedness.

syndactyly a fusion of fingers or toes which is a CONGENITAL effect. It may affect two or more fingers through webbing, or result in complete fusion of all digits.

syndrome a number of symptoms and signs that together constitute a particular condition.

synovial fluid see SYNOVIAL MEMBRANE.

synovial membrane (or **synovium**) the inner membrane of a capsule that encloses a joint that moves freely. It secretes into the joint a thick lubricating fluid (synovial fluid) which may build up after injury to cause pain.

synovitis inflammation of the SYNOVIAL MEMBRANE that lines a joint capsule. The result is swelling with pain. It is associated with rheumatic disease, injury or infection (e.g. chronic tuberculosis). The treatment depends upon the cause of the condition and often a sample of the synovial fluid is taken for examination.

syphilis an infectious, sexually-transmitted disease, caused by the bacterium *Treponema pallidum* which shows symptoms in three stages. Bacteria enter the body through mucous membranes during sexual intercourse and an ulcer appears in the first instance. Within a short time the LYMPH NODES locally and then all over the body enlarge and harden and this lasts several weeks.

Secondary symptoms appear about two months after infection and include fever, pains, enlarged lymph nodes and a faint rash which is usually noticed on the chest. The bacterium is found in enormous numbers in the primary sores and any skin lesions of the secondary stage. The final stage may not appear until many months or years after infection and comprises the formation of numerous tumour-like masses throughout the body (in skin, muscle, bone, brain, spinal cord and other organs such as the liver, stomach. etc.). This stage can cause serious damage to the heart, brain or spinal cod resulting in blindness, TABES DORSALIS, and mental disability.

CONGENITAL syphilis is much rarer than the former, *acquired*, type. It is contracted by a developing foetus from the mother and symptoms show a few weeks after birth. Treatment of syphilis is with penicillin early in the development of the disease.

systemic general term referring to the body as a whole.

systole the contraction of the heart that alternates with the resting phase (diastole). It usually refers to ventricular systole which at 0.3 seconds is three times longer than atrial systole.

systolic pressure *see* BLOOD PRESSURE.

T

tachycardia increased rate of heart beat which may be caused naturally as with exercise or be symptomatic of disease.

talus the ankle bone which articulates with the lower leg bones (TIBIA and FIBULA) above and also with the heel bone (*calcaneus*) below (*see* TARSUS).

tampon a plug of compressed gause inserted into a wound or cavity to absorb blood.

tarsus a part of the foot in the region

of the instep consisting of seven bones, chiefly the TALUS and the *calcaneus* (heel bone) and also the cuboid, navicular and three cuneiform bones.

taste the perception of flavour brought about by CHEMORECEPTORS (the TASTE BUDS) situated on the tongue.

taste buds the sensory receptors responsible for the perception of taste, located in the grooves around the papillae of the TONGUE, in the epiglottis, parts of the PHARYNX and soft palate. The taste buds are stimulated by the presence of dissolved food in the saliva and messages are sent via nerves to the brain where the information is interpreted and perceived.

taxis the returning to their normal position of displaced organs, parts of organs or bones by manipulation (*see* HERNIA).

teeth *see* TOOTH.

temperature (of the body) the normal body temperature is around 37°C (98.4°F) but it varies considerably both between individuals and in one person throughout the day. In addition, temperature differences occur between various areas of the body being lower in the skin than internally.

temple the side of the head above the level of the eye and the ear.

temporal one of the main areas of the CEREBRAL CORTEX in each of the CEREBRAL HEMISPHERES of the brain, occurring in the TEMPORAL region of the skull. A cleft known as the *lateral sulcus* separates it from the frontal lobe.

temporal lobe epilepsy EPILEPSY which is centred within the temporal lobe caused by disease within the cortex. It is characterized by hallucinations involving the senses of taste, smell, hearing and sight and memory disturbances. During an attack, the person usually remains conscious but not fully and normally aware, and afterwards may not have any memory of what has occurred.

tendinitis inflammation of a tendon which often results from excessive or unaccustomed exercise but may also result from infection.

tendon a tough and inelastic white cord composed of bundles of COLLAGEN fibres which attaches a muscle to a bone. A tendon concentrates the pull of the muscle onto one point on the bone and the length and thickness varies considerably. The fibres of a tendon pass into, and become continuous with, those of the bone it serves. Many tendons are enclosed in tendon sheaths lined with SYNOVIAL MEMBRANE containing synovial fluid which reduces friction and enables easy movement to occur.

tennis elbow a form of TENDINITIS affecting the tendon at the outer part of the elbow which becomes inflamed and painful.

teratogen a substance or disease or any other factor which causes the production of abnormalities in a foetus. The drugs in this category include thalidomide and alcohol. German measles and cytomegalovirus are among the infections.

teratogenesis the processes which result in the development of physical abnormalities in a foetus.

teratoma a tumour that is composed of unusual tissues not normally found at that site and derived from partially developed embryological cells. Teratomas are most common in the ovary and testicle (particularly if latter undescended).

testicle (testis) one of the pair of male sex organs situated within the SCROTUM which produce spermatozoa and secrete the hormone TESTOSTERONE. The testicles develop within the abdomen of the foetus but descend around the time of birth into the scrotum.

Each testicle has an outer double membrane layer known as the *tunica vaginalis*. The tunica vaginalis contains an inner fibrous layer called the *tunica albuginea* which protects the testicle. The bulk of the testicle consists of numerous fine, convoluted tubules called seminiferous tubules which are lined with cells that produce the spermatozoa. In addition, other cells known as *sertoli cells*, occur which provide support and possibly nourishment for the developing spermatozoa. The tubules are supported by connective tissue containing nerves and blood vessels and also the *cells of Leydig* which are responsible for hormone production. The tubules connect with another highly folded tube called the *epididymis* which is about 7m long and connects with the VAS DEFERENS which leads to the URETHRA. The spermatozoa are passed by passive movement along the epididymis, completing their development as they go and are stored in the lower part until EJACULATION.

testis *see* TESTICLE.

testosterone the male sex hormone secreted by the TESTES (*see also* ANDROGEN).

tetanus a very serious and sometimes fatal infectious disease, the non-medical name for which is *lockjaw*.

It is caused by the bacterium *Clostridium tetani*, spores of which enter through a wound. Rapid multiplication of the bacteria produces a toxin which affects the nerves resulting in rigidity and spasm of muscles. Often there is high fever and the spasms cause extreme agony.

If respiratory muscles are involved death may occur by asphyxia.

thalamus one of a pair of masses of grey matter located within each side of the forebrain. Each is a centre for coordinating and relaying sensory information concerned with all the senses apart from that of smell.

thalidomide a TERATOGENIC drug which was formerly prescribed for treatment of MORNING SICKNESS in pregnancy. It was withdrawn when it was discovered that it caused developmental damage to the foetus, particularly malformation of limbs.

therapeutics the area of medicine concerned with the various methods of healing and treatment.

therapy the treatment of disease.

thermography a method of recording the heat produced by different areas of the body using photographic film sensitive to infrared radiation. Areas with good blood circulation produce more heat and this can occur abnormally if a tumour is present. The record thus obtained is a *thermogram* and this is one of the techniques used to detect breast tumours (*mammothermography*).

thiamine *see* VITAMIN B.

Thiersch's graft a type of skin graft in which thin strips of skin, involving the epidermis and the upper layer of the dermis, are taken from one part of the body and placed on the wound which requires to be healed.

thigh the part of the leg above the knee.

thoracocentesis also known as *pleuracentesis*. The withdrawal, by means of a hollow needle inserted through the chest wall, of fluid from the pleural cavity.

thorax the chest.

thrombin an enzyme derived from prothrombin, its inactive precursor, which is formed and is active during the final stages of blood clotting (*see* COAGULATION).

thromboembolism the situation in which a blood clot (THROMBUS) forms in one part of the circulation, usually a vein in the leg (phlebothrombosis), and a portion breaks off and becomes lodged elsewhere causing a total blockage (EMBOLISM). The embolism often involves the pulmonary artery or one of its branches and this is known as PULMONARY EMBOLISM.

thrombolysis the dissolving of blood clots by enzyme activity. Natural enzymes produced within the body have this effect but drug treatment, especially involving streptokinase, may be used to break up clots following PULMONARY EMBOLISM, CORONARY THROMBOSIS and PHLEBOTHROMBOSIS.

thrombophlebitis inflammation of the wall of a vein along with clot formation in the affected section of the vessel.

This is a complication of pregnancy and may be dangerous, involving a deep vein thrombosis which can result in PULMONARY EMBOLISM.

thrombosis the process of clotting within a blood vessel producing a THROMBUS. It may occur within an artery or vein, often one which is dis-

eased or damaged, and can be very serious or even fatal, e.g. STROKE, CORONARY THROMBOSIS.

thrombus a blood clot within a vessel which partially or totally obstructs the circulation.

thrush an infection caused by the fungus *Candida albicans* which affects the mucous membranes of the mouth and vagina producing white patches. It is a popular name given to a group of infections known as *candidiasis*.

thymus a gland, divided into two lobes, which is present in the neck and which forms a vital part of the immune system. It is especially large in children and important in the development of the immune response and the production of lymphoid tissue. After puberty, the thymus gradually begins to shrink. Bone marrow cells, known as *stem cells*, undergo maturation within the thymus and one group, the *T. lymphocytes*, are dependent upon the gland. These are very important cells in the body which produce ANTIBODIES.

thyroidectomy surgical removal of the thyroid gland.

thyroid gland a bilobed endocrine gland situated at the base and front of the neck. It is enclosed by fibrous tissue and well-supplied with blood, and internally consists of numerous vesicles containing a jelly-like colloidal substance. These vesicles produce thyroid hormone, which is rich in iodine, under the control of *thyroid stimulating hormone* (THYROTROPHIN STIMULATING HORMONE) released from the PITUITARY GLAND. Two hormones are produced by the gland, thyroxine and triiodothyronine, which are essential for the regulation of metabolism and growth. *See also* CRETINISM, MYXOEDEMA and HYPERTHYROIDISM.

thyrotoxic adenoma a form of THYRO-TOXICOSIS or GRAVES' DISEASE.

thyrotoxicosis *see* GRAVES' DISEASE.

thyrotrophin releasing hormone a hormone produced and released from the HYPOTHALAMUS which acts on the anterior lobe of the PITUITARY GLAND which then releases THYROTROPHIN STIMULATING HORMONE (*see* THYROID).

thyrotrophin stimulating hormone a hormone produced and released by the anterior pituitary gland which stimulates the THYROID GLAND to produce its hormones (*see* THYROID).

thyroxine an important hormone produced by the thyroid gland and used medically to treat conditions resulting from underactivity of this gland, e.g. CRETINISM and MYXOEDEMA.

tibia the larger of the two bones in the lower leg known as the shin bone articulating above with the FEMUR and with the TALUS of the ankle below.

tinnitus any ringing or buzzing sound in the ear which does not have a real external cause. Many disorders of the ear can cause this, for example, hardened wax, Ménière's disease, drugs including aspirin and quinine, and damage to the auditory nerve. In many cases no underlying cause is found.

tolerance the adaptation of the body to a particular drug or substance so that over a period of time, there is a reduction in the response to a particular dose. Usually a larger dose must now be given to produce the same effect as before.

tomography a particular technique using X-rays or ultrasound so that structures at a given depth are brought into sharp focus while those at other levels are deliberately blurred. In this way, pictures of *slices* of the body are obtained at different levels to build up a three-dimensional image. The image obtained is called a *tomogram*.

tongue the muscular and highly mobile organ attached to the floor of the mouth, the three main functions of which are manipulation of food during chewing prior to swallowing, taste and production of speech. The three areas of the tongue are the tip, body and root and it is covered with a mucous membrane which unites with that of the mouth and pharynx.

The tongue is anchored at the root by various muscles which attach it to the back of the mouth. In addition, the undersurface of the tongue is attached in the midline to the floor of the mouth by a fold of mucous membrane called the *frenulum lingae*. If this is attached too far forward to restrict the movement at the tip it causes the condition known as *tongue tie*.

The surface is covered with minute projections called papillae, of which there are three different kinds, filiform, fungiform and circumvallate. There are grooves surrounding the papillae in which the TASTE BUDS occur. The tongue is well supplied with blood and receives branches from five different nerves on each side.

tonsillectomy surgical removal of the TONSILS.

tonsillitis inflammation of the tonsils caused by bacterial or viral infection. The symptoms include a severe sore throat causing painful swallowing, accompanied by fever and earache, especially in children. The tonsils are swollen and white in appearance due to infected material exuded from them and glands in the neck are enlarged.

tonsils usually refers to the two small masses of lymphoid tissue situated on either side at the back of the mouth (the *palatine tonsils*). However, another pair occur below the tongue which are the *lingual tonsils* while the ADENOIDS are the PHARYNGEAL TONSILS. All are part of the body's protective mechanism against infection.

tooth a hard structure used for biting and chewing. Each tooth consists of a *root* embedded in a socket within the jawbone to which it is attached by the fibrous *periodontal membrane*. The projecting part of the tooth is called the *crown* which is covered with a hard resistant layer of *enamel*, (composed primarily of calcium phosphate and calcium carbonate). The root is covered with a thin hard layer of cementum.

Most of the interior of the tooth consists of *dentine*, a hard ivory-like substance which surrounds the inner core or pulp. The pulp contains blood vessels and nerve fibres and is connected with the dentine by means of fine cellular processes. There are four different types of teeth, canine, incisor, premolar and molar.

torpor a state of physical and mental sluggishness which accompanies various mental disorders, some kinds of poisoning and may be present in elderly people with arterial disease.

torsion twisting, often referring to an abnormal state of the whole or part of an organ which impairs the nerve and blood supply. Examples are a torsion of a loop of bowel or of the spermatic cord of the testicle. Surgery is usually required to correct a torsion.

touch the sense which is conferred by specialized sensory receptors present in the skin (and also in muscles and other areas of the body), which enable sensations of pain, temperature, pressure and touch to be perceived. The sense organs involved are specially adapted to respond to particular sensations conveying their messages to the brain along different nerve pathways.

tourniquet a device used to arrest bleeding, usually from an artery in a limb, which may be a length of bandage, rubber tube or cord tied tightly round generally as an emergency measure. Direct pressure on a wound is now considered to be preferable as a first aid measure, because a tourniquet can deprive all the tissues of oxygen by arresting the circulation, and there is a risk of damage and of gangrene.

toxaemia blood poisoning resulting from the toxins produced by rapidly multiplying bacteria at a localized site of infection such as an abscess. Symptoms are varied including fever, vomiting and diarrhoea and a general feeling of being unwell. The source of the infection has to be treated with antibiotic drugs. Toxaemia of pregnancy involves two relatively rare conditions known as ECLAMPSIA and PRE-ECLAMPSIA.

toxicology the scientific study of poisons and their effects.

toxic shock syndrome a state of acute

shock due to SEPTICAEMIA and caused by toxins produced by *staphylococcal* bacteria. The symptoms include high fever, skin rash and diarrhoea and can prove rapidly fatal if not adequately treated with antibiotics, especially PENICILLIN and *cephalosporin*, along with fluid and salt replacement.

The syndrome is associated with the use of tampons by women during menstruation, particularly if a tampon is left in place too long. However, the syndrome can also occur in other people and is in all cases rare.

toxin a poison produced by bacteria and by many species of plant and also present in snake venom. In the body, a toxin acts as an ANTIGEN and provokes the production of special antibodies called antitoxins. The antitoxins produced may be used in IMMUNIZATION to protect against the disease as with tetanus and diphtheria. An *endotoxin* is contained within the bacterial cell and only released when the organism dies and decays. Endotoxins do not provoke antitoxin production (*see* TOXOID).

toxocariasis a disease caused by the larvae of roundworms which normally infect the domestic dog (*Toxicara canis*) and cat (*Toxicara cati*), but can be passed to man by swallowing material contaminated with eggs in infected faeces.

Those most at risk are children, especially at a young age when hands may become infected while playing. Once swallowed, the larvae which hatch from the eggs travel around the body in the circulation and can cause considerable damage to, for example, the lungs and liver. Also,

the larvae may lodge in the retina of the eye causing inflammation and the production of abnormal granulated tissue called granuloma.

Symptoms of the infection include muscular pain, fever, skin rash, respiratory problems, vomiting and convulsions. Treatment is with drugs, such as diethylcarbamazine and thiabendazole.

toxoid a preparation of TOXIN which has been treated with chemicals so that it cannot cause disease but is able to provoke the production of antitoxin. This is the basis of VACCINES against diphtheria and tetanus.

toxoplasmosis an infectious disease caused by a protozoan organism known as *Toxoplasma*. The infection is either transmitted by eating undercooked meat or through direct contact with contaminated soil or especially with infected cats. This form of the infection is mild and causes few ill effects. However, a much more serious form of the disease can be passed from a mother infected during pregnancy to her unborn baby. The newborn infant may suffer from HYDROCEPHALUS, mental retardation, blindness or may even be stillborn. Treatment is by means of sulphonamide drugs and pyrimethamine.

tracer a substance which is marked so that when it is introduced into the body its progress can be followed e.g. radioactive tracers used in the detection of brain tumours and thyroid disease.

trachea the windpipe which is the part of the air passage that is situated between the LARYNX and the bronchi.

tracheitis inflammation of the trachea, often accompanying a viral infection of the upper respiratory tract. The symptoms include a persistent painful cough and sore chest and it often accompanies BRONCHITIS and also DIPHTHERIA.

tracheostomy (*or* **tracheotomy**) a surgical procedure in which a hole is made in the trachea to allow direct access of air to the lower respiratory passages. This may be performed in an emergency if there is an obstruction in breathing. However, usually this operation is carried out in hospital, especially on patients in intensive therapy who require long-term artificial ventilation. This is to avoid the damage to the trachea which is caused by the long-term use of an endotracheal breathing tube (inserted through the nose or mouth) which would normally be used first.

Once the opening has been made a double tube is inserted and held in place by tapes around the neck. The inner tube can be freely withdrawn and replaced and needs to be kept scrupulously clean and free from any obstruction.

traction the use of weights and pulleys to apply a pulling force on a broken bone, to ensure that it is kept correctly aligned while healing takes place.

trance a sleep-like state in which a person ceases to react normally to the environment and loses the power of voluntary movement, but remains aware. It can be induced by HYPNOSIS, meditation, hysteria, CATATONIA and drug abuse.

tranquillizer a drug that has a soothing and calming effect, relieving stress and anxiety. Minor tranquillizers such as diazepam and chlordiazepoxide are widely used to relieve these symptoms which may arise from a variety of causes. There is a danger of dependence with long-term use. Major tranquillizers e.g. chlorpromazine and haloperidol are used to treat severe mental illnesses such as SCHIZOPHRENIA.

transfusion *see* BLOOD TRANSFUSION.

transplantation the transfer of an organ or tissue from one person to another (*called an allotransplant*) or within the body of an individual (*autotransplant*). It undermeaningly refers to skin and bone GRAFTING. The person from whom the organ is obtained is known as the *donor* and the one who receives it is known as the *recipient*.

Organ transplants involving the kidney, heart, bone marrow, cornea, lungs and liver have all become more common.

trauma an event which causes physical damage such as a fracture or an emotional shock brought about by a harmful and upsetting circumstance.

travel sickness *see* MOTION SICKNESS.

tremor involuntary movements which may involve the whole of a muscle or only part of it and produce fine trembling or more pronounced shaking. Tremors are classified according to the type of movement produced and are a symptom of many diseases including CHOREA, MULTIPLE SCLEROSIS and PARKINSONISM.

trench fever an infectious disease caused by *Rickettsia quintana* which was epidemic among troops in the First World War and still occurs in Mexico. It is transmitted to man by the body louse and causes fever, rash, leg aches and general weakness.

triceps a three-headed muscle present in the upper arm which extends the forearm.

trichomoniasis two types of infection caused by a protozoan organism which either attacks the digestive system causing DYSENTERY (*Trichomonas hominis*), or causes vaginal inflammation and discharge (*Trichomonas vaginalis*). In the latter case the infection can be transmitted to a male sexual partner. The drug metronidazole is highly effective.

trichorrhoea the medical name for the falling out of hair which may be due to disease such as typhoid fever or scarlet fever or have no apparent cause.

tricuspid valve a valve with three flaps or cusps that controls the passage of blood from the right ATRIUM to the right VENTRICLE of the heart and normally prevents backflow (*see* HEART).

trigeminal nerve the fifth and largest of the cranial nerves which has three divisions, the *mandibular, maxillary* and *ophthalmic* nerves. The ophthalmic and maxillary are sensory nerves and the mandibular has both sensory and motor functions. Hence the trigeminal nerve is involved in the relaying and perception of sensations (temperature, touch, pain, etc.) from the whole of the face and mouth and also in controlling the muscles involved in chewing.

trigeminal neuralgia also known as Tic Doulourex. This is a severe form of NEURALGIA which can affect all the divisions of the trigeminal nerve. It affects women more commonly than men, especially those over the age of 50. It causes severe pain of a burning or cutting nature which can be constant or spasmodic and may be provoked by simple actions such as eating or by heat or cold. The skin of the face may be inflamed and the eye red and watery and the neuralgia is usually confined to one side. The condition is debilitating in that the pain is so intense and interferes with sleeping and eating but the drug carbamazepine is proving to be highly beneficial.

triglycerides fats consisting of three fatty acid molecules combined with glycerol which are the form in which the body stores fat. Triglycerides are derived from the digestion of fats in food.

trophic a term referring to nutrition, e.g. trophic fracture which occurs when the bone is weakened due to poor nourishment in the person concerned.

truss a device consisting of a pad attached to a belt with spring straps to maintain its position, which is worn under clothing to support a HERNIA.

trypanosomiasis *see* SLEEPING SICKNESS.

trypsin an important enzyme involved in the digestion of proteins. Its inactive precursor, trypsinogen, is secreted by the PANCREAS and converted to trypsin in the DUODENUM by the action of another enzyme called enteropeptidase.

tubercle either a small rounded knob on a bone e.g. on the ribs or a minute nodular tissue mass (lesion) which is characteristic of TUBERCULOSIS.

tuberculosis a group of infections caused by the bacillus (bacterium) *Mycobacterium tuberculosis* of which pulmonary tuberculosis of the lungs (consumption or phthisis) is the best known form. The pulmonary disease is acquired through inhalation of air containing the organism from an infected person, or dust laden with bacteria. People infected in this way can show no symptoms but still be carriers. In the lungs, the infection causes formation of a *primary tubercle* which spreads to lymph nodes to form the *primary complex*.

The disease may wax and wane for years as the body's natural immune system acts against the infection. If the infection is severe, symptoms include fever, wasting, night sweats and the coughing up of blood. The bacteria may enter the blood stream and spread throughout the body setting up numerous tubercles in other tissues (*miliary tuberculosis*). The disease is curable with antibiotics, e.g. streptomycin. In addition, BCG VACCINATION as a preventive measure is given to children in the UK, in addition to X-ray screening to detect carriers.

tumour any abnormal swelling occurring in any part of the body consisting of an unusual growth of tissue and which may be malignant or benign. Tumours tend to be classified according to the tissue of which they are composed, e.g. FIBROMA (mainly fibrous tissue) and MYOMA (largely muscle fibres).

turgor a state of being distended, engorged or swollen.

Turner's syndrome a genetic disorder affecting females in which there is only one X chromosome instead of the usual two. Hence those af-fected have 45 instead of 46 chromosomes, are infertile (as the ovaries are absent), menstruation is absent and breasts and body hair do not develop. Those affected are short, may have webbing of the neck and other developmental defects. The heart may be affected and there can be deafness and intellectual impairment. In a less severe form of the disorder, the second X chromosome is present but abnormal, lacking in normal genetic material.

tympanic membrane the eardrum which separates the middle and outer ears and which vibrates in response to sound waves transmitting the vibrations to one of the ear ossicles (the *malleus*). *See* EAR.

typhoid fever a severe infectious disease of the digestive system which is caused by the bacterium *Salmonella typhi* and causes symptoms including a rise in temperature, a rash on the abdomen and chest, headache and nosebleeds. The temperature rise occurs in a characteristic fashion known as a *stepladder temperature*. In severe cases there may be ulceration of the intestinal wall leading to PERITONITIS if an ulcer bursts, or haemorrhage from the bowels and inflammation of the lungs, SPLEEN and bones. In these cases the disease can prove to be fatal. The infection is acquired through ingesting contaminated food or water hence preventive measures involving high standards of hygiene and sanitation are important.

typhus fever *see* RICKETTSIAE.

U

ulcer a break on the skin surface or on the MUCOUS MEMBRANE lining within the body cavities that may be inflamed and fails to heal. Ulcers of the skin include BEDSORES and varicose ulcers (which are caused by defective circulation). For ulcers of the alimentary tract, *see* DUODENAL ULCER, GASTRIC ULCER and PEPTIC ULCER.

ulna one of the two bones making up the forearm. It is the inner and longer of the two bones (the other being the radius). It articulates with the radius at both ends and additionally with the humerus above, and indirectly with the wrist below.

ultrasound (*or* **ultrasonic waves**) high frequency sound waves (above 20 kHz), beyond the range of the human ear. Ultrasound is used to examine the body's organs, ducts, etc. in addition to assessing the progress of a developing foetus. The patient is not submitted to harmful radiation as with other techniques and no contrast medium is required. It can be used to examine the liver, kidney, bladder, pancreas, ovaries and is used in diagnosing brain tumours. The vibrations of the sound waves can be used in other ways, e.g. breaking up kidney stones.

umbilical cord the cord connecting the foetus to the placenta, containing two arteries and one vein. It is approximately 60cm long and after birth it is severed and the stump shrivels to leave a scar, the navel or UMBILICUS.

umbilicus the navel (*see* UMBILICAL CORD).

unconsciousness the state of being partially or totally unaware of the surroundings and lacking in response to stimuli. Sleep is a natural form of unconsciousness. Unnatural states of unconsciousness can be due to numerous causes including injuries to the brain resulting in compression or concussion, fainting due to insufficient blood supply to the brain, EPILEPSY, poisoning and various diseases, e.g. DIABETES MELLITUS.

undulant fever *see* BRUCELLOSIS.

ungual a term meaning relating to the fingernails or toenails.

unguentum the term in pharmacy for an ointment.

unguis a fingernail or toenail.

uraemia the condition where there is excess UREA in the blood due to kidney disease or failure. Waste products are usually excreted by the kidneys but accumulation in the blood leads to headaches, drowsiness and lethargy, nausea and vomiting and diarrhoea. Eventually, without treatment, death follows. Haemodialysis on a kidney machine may be necessary or even a renal transplant.

urataemia the presence in the blood of urate compounds (*see* URIC ACID), associated with GOUT, when urates are deposited in the body.

urea a metabolic byproduct of the chemical breakdown of protein and the form in which excess nitrogen is removed from the body, in urine. It is formed in the LIVER and taken in the blood to the KIDNEYS. The amount excreted daily is 30–35gm. Although urea is not poisonous in itself, an excess in the blood (URAEMIA) implies a defective kidney which will cause an excess of other waste products that may be poisonous.

ureaplasma microorganisms responsible for diseases such as PROSTATITIS, nonspecific URETHRITIS and infertility and NEONATAL death. The latter can be associated with infection of the placenta by *Ureaplasma urealyticum*.

ureter the tubes joining the KIDNEYS to the bladder and through which urine passes. The muscular ureter walls contract to force urine into the bladder.

ureterectomy surgical excision of a URETER, usually with the removal of the associated kidney.

ureteritis inflammation of the URETER which usually occurs with bladder inflammations.

ureteroenterostomy the creation by surgery of a link between the URETER and the bowel, thus bypassing the bladder. The join is made at the SIGMOID COLON and is made to bypass a diseased bladder. The urine is then passed with the faeces, thus avoiding an external opening for collection of urine.

ureteroplasty reconstruction of a damaged or diseased ureter by surgery, using bowel or bladder tissue.

ureteroscope an instrument introduced into a dilated URETER often to locate a stone or remove stone fragments created by ultrasonic destruction of a larger stone.

ureterostomy the creation of an external opening to the URETER whereby the ureter is brought to the surface to permit drainage.

ureterotomy an incision into the URETER, commonly to remove a stone.

urethra the duct carrying urine from the bladder out of the body. It is about 3.5cm long in women and 20cm in men. The male urethra runs through the penis and also forms the ejaculatory duct.

urethritis inflammation of the mucous lining of the URETHRA which may be associated with CYSTITIS, often being the cause of the latter. The commonest cause of urethritis is GONORRHOEA (*specific* urethritis). Alternatively, it may be due to infection with microorganisms (causing *nonspecific* urethritis). The symptoms include a discharge, pain on passing urine, and inflammations in other organs such as the bladder and testicle are possible. Sulphonamide and antibiotic drugs are effective, once the infecting organism is identified.

uric acid an organic acid that contains nitrogen and is the end-product of the metabolism of protein. It occurs in the urine but in small amounts (less than 1gm). It is formed in the liver and excreted by the kidneys but in excess, salts (urates) form and occur as stone in the urinary tract. Deposits of urates in joints is a feature of GOUT.

urinary organs the system responsible for the extraction of components from the blood to form urine, its storage and periodic discharge from the body. The organs are the kidneys, ureters, bladder and urethra (*see individual entries*).

urinary tract the system of ducts that permit movement of urine out of the body from the kidneys, i.e. the URE-TERS, BLADDER and URETHRA.

urination (*or* **micturition**) the discharge of urine from the body via the URETHRA. It is begun by a voluntary relaxation of the sphincter muscle below the bladder.

urine the body's fluid waste excreted by the KIDNEYS. The waste products include UREA, URIC ACID and creatinine (produced by muscles) with salt, phosphates and sulphates and ammonia also present. In a solution with about 95-96% water, there may be 100 or more compounds but the vast majority occur only in trace amounts. Many diseases alter the quantity and composition of urine and its analysis is standard procedure to assist diagnosis of diseases.

urine retention the condition when urine is produced by the kidneys but it is retained in the bladder. This may be due to an obstruction, or a weakness in the bladder. Enlargement of the PROSTATE GLAND is a common cause of blockage. It may also be caused by a STRICTURE due to injury scar or ulceration.

urinogenital a collective descriptive term relating to all organs and tissues involved in excretion and reproduction, because they are closely linked anatomically and functionally.

urology the subdiscipline of medicine dealing with diseases of the urinary tract, from the kidney to the urethra.

urticaria (*or* **nettle rash**) an allergic reaction by an individual to some substance to which they are hypersensitive, in which the allergic response is manifested on the skin. Raised red patches develop which may last for hours or days. There is intense itching.

The sensitivity may be to certain foods, e.g. shellfish, and the effect may occur anywhere on the body, but commonly erupts on the face and trunk. If it also affects the tongue or throat, there is danger of a blockage of the airway which would need urgent attention.

uterine relating to the UTERUS.

uterus (*or* **womb**) a vaguely pear-shaped organ within the cavity of the pelvis that is specialized for the growth and nourishment of a foetus. FALLOPIAN TUBES connect to the upper part and the lower part joins the VAGINA at the CERVIX. It has a plentiful blood supply with lymphatic vessels and nerves. During pregnancy it enlarges considerably and the SMOOTH MUSCLE walls thicken. Contractions of the muscular wall push the foetus out via the vagina at childbirth. If there is no pregnancy the lining undergoes periodic changes (MENSTRUATION).

uvea the middle pigmented layer of the EYE consisting of the IRIS, choroid and ciliary body.

uveitis inflammation of any part of the uvea. The iris and ciliary body are often both inflamed (*anterior uveitis*) producing a painful condition, unlike *posterior uveitis* (when the choroid is affected).

V

vaccination the production of immunity to a disease by inoculation with a VACCINE or a specially prepared material that stimulates the production of antibodies.

vaccine a modified preparation of a BACTERIUM or VIRUS that is no longer dangerous but will stimulate development of antibodies and therefore confer immunity against actual infection with the disease. Other vaccines consist of specific toxins (e.g. tetanus), or dead bacteria (e.g. cholera and typhoid). Live but weakened organisms are used against smallpox and tuberculosis.

vagina the lower part of the female reproductive tract that leads from the uterus to the exterior. It receives the erect penis during sexual intercourse. The semen is ejaculated into the upper part from where the sperms pass through the CERVIX and UTERUS to the FALLOPIAN TUBES. The vagina is a muscular tube lined with mucous membrane.

vaginismus a sudden and painful contraction of muscles surrounding the VAGINA in response to contact of the vagina or VULVA, e.g. an attempted intercourse. It may be due to a fear of intercourse or an inflammation.

vaginitis inflammation of the vagina due to infection or deficiency in diet, or hygiene. There may be itching, a discharge and pain on urination.

vagotomy the cutting of fibres of the VAGUS nerve to the stomach. The operation can be performed to reduce the stomach's acid and pepsin secretion, in treatment of a PEPTIC ULCER.

vagus the tenth cranial nerve which comprises motor, sensory, vasodilator and secretory fibres. It supplies the muscles for swallowing and fibres go to the heart, throat, lungs and stomach and other organs in the abdomen. It also carries the taste sensation from the mouth.

valve a structure within an organ or vessel that restricts flow to one direction, whether the fluid be blood or lymph. The valves comprise cusps on the vessel wall. The cusp is like a membranous pocket that fills with blood should it flow back and the cusps distend and close the valve.

valvular heart disease affects mainly the AORTIC and MITRAL VALVES which may narrow (STENOSIS) or weaken. Aortic valve disease is associated more with old age while mitral valve disease is rheumatic in origin.

valvotomy an operation undertaken to open a stenosed heart valve and render it functional. Several techniques are available including surgery, an inflating balloon or a dilating instrument.

valvulitis inflammation of a valve, particularly in the heart. It is commonly due to rheumatic fever.

varicose veins veins that have become stretched, distended and twisted. The superficial veins in the legs are often affected although it may occur elsewhere. Causes include congenitally defective valves, obesity, pregnancy and THROMBOPHLEBITIS (inflammation of the wall of a vein with secondary THROMBOSIS in the affected part of the vein). Elastic support is a common treatment although alternatives are SCLEROTHERAPY and PHLEBECTOMY.

variola a name for SMALLPOX.

vas a vessel or duct, especially those carrying blood, lymph or spermatozoa.

vascular relating to blood vessels; supplied with blood vessels.

vasculitis inflammation of the blood vessels that may cause damage to the linings and cause narrowing. It may result from several conditions including acute NEPHRITIS and SERUM SICKNESS.

vas deferens (*plural* **vas deferentia**) one of the two tubes that join the testes to the ejaculatory duct via the PROSTATE GLAND. It carries spermatozoa to the URETHRA on ejaculation, aided by contraction of its muscular wall.

vasectomy the cutting of the VAS DEFERENS, which is performed on both ducts causing sterility, although the effect is not immediate.

vasoconstriction the narrowing of blood vessels with a consequent reduction in blood supply to that part of the body supplied. A variety of circumstances can cause vasoconstriction including cold and shock.

vasodilation (**vasodilatation**) the increase in diameter of blood vessels lowering blood pressure.

vasopressin (**antidiuretic hormone**) a PITUITARY GLAND hormone that con-

stricts blood vessels and reduces urine secretion by increasing the water reabsorbed by the KIDNEY.

vasovagal attack fainting, precipitated by a slowing of the heart and a fall in blood pressure. This may be due to shock, severe pain, fear, etc. and is caused by excessive stimulation of the VAGUS nerve which participates in the control of breathing and the circulation.

vasovasostomy the reversal of VASECTOMY.

vector commonly an insect that carries parasitic microorganisms between people, or from animals to people, e.g. mosquitoes carrying malaria.

vein one of the numerous blood vessels carrying deoxygenated blood to the right atrium of the heart (the one exception is the PULMONARY vein). Each vein has three tissue layers, similar to the layers of the heart. Veins are less elastic than arteries and collapse when cut. They also contain VALVES to prevent backflow.

vena cava either of two major veins carrying blood from other veins to the right ATRIUM of the heart. The *inferior* vena cava takes blood from the body below the DIAPHRAGM and the *superior* vena cava takes blood from the head, neck, arms and thorax.

venereal disease (*or* **sexually transmitted disease**) a disease transmitted by sexual intercourse. This includes AIDS, SYPHILIS, GONORRHOEA, nonspecific URETHRITIS, etc.

venography examination of veins using X-rays after injection of a radio-opaque substance. This enables leaks, blockages or other abnormalities to be identified.

venom the poisonous substance produced by snakes, scorpions, etc. which in humans may produce only localized pain and swelling, or in serious cases cause more general effects and even death.

ventilation the means whereby air passes into and out of the lungs, aided by movement of the diaphragm.

Artificial ventilation is the use of a machine (VENTILATOR) to regulate a person's breathing. This may occur during an operation. Also, damage to the relevant part of the brain, chest injury, lung disease or nerve and muscle disorders may all require the use of artificial ventilation.

ventilator the machine used to provide an air supply to the lungs of patients who cannot breathe normally for themselves. Blood gases and other body functions can be monitored at the same time.

ventouse (*or* **vacuum extractor**) a machine used in childbirth, comprising a suction cup attached to the head of the foetus enabling it to be gently pulled out of the uterus. It is an alternative to the use of forceps.

ventricle one of the two major chambers within the heart. They are thick-walled and muscular and form the main pumping chamber. The right ventricle receives blood from the right ATRIUM and venae cavae and its outflow is the PULMONARY artery. The left ventricle takes blood from the pulmonary vein via the left atrium, and its outflow is the AORTA.

Also cavities within the brain, filled with cerebrospinal fluid.

ventricular fibrillation a dangerous rapid ARRHYTHMIA of the ventricle.

verruca a term for WART.

verrucose covered with warts.

version also known as *turning*, the procedure to move a foetus in the uterus to a more normal position, to make delivery easier.

vertebra (*plural* **vertebrae**) any of the bones making up the vertebral column. Each has a cavity (the vertebral canal or foramen) and various processes for attachment of muscles or articulation of adjacent vertebrae. The spinal cord passes through the vertebral canal (*see* SPINAL COLUMN).

vertebral column *see* SPINAL COLUMN.

vertigo a condition in which a person has a false sensation of imbalance and of the surroundings moving. It is commonly a sensation of spinning but may be as if the ground is tilting. The semicircular canals of the ear are fundamental in the maintenance of balance and vertigo is generally due to some problem with this mechanism or with the appropriate centres in the brain.

vesicular breathing soft, normal sounds of breathing heard in the lung by means of a stethoscope. The sounds change when the lungs are diseased and the different sounds help a doctor diagnose the disease.

vessel any tube that carries fluid, particularly blood or lymph.

vestigial the term applied to an organ that has progressively, over a long time, lost its function and structure to become rudimentary.

viable able to liver separately.

villus (*plural* **villi**) *see* JEJUNUM.

Vincent's angina a former name for ulcerative gingivitis and ulcerative inflammation of the throat, caused by bacteria.

viral haemorrhagic fever a viral disease with a high mortality rate. After the incubation period there is headache, fever, severe internal bleeding, diarrhoea and vomiting. Death may follow, usually eight or nine days later. Serum taken from someone recovering from the disease is a useful source of antibodies.

viral pneumonia an acute lung infection caused by one of many viruses. The symptoms include fever, headache, muscle pains and a thick sputum associated with the cough. It often occurs after a viral infection and treatment, in the main, deals with the symptoms only.

virology the study of viruses.

virulence the ability of a bacterium of virus to cause disease, measured by numbers of people infected, the speed with which it spreads.

virus the smallest microbe that is completely parasitic, because it is only capable of replication within the cells of its host. Viruses infect animals, plants and microorganisms. Viruses are classified according to their NUCLEIC ACIDS and can contain double or single-stranded DNA or RNA. In an infection the virus binds to the host cells and then penetrates the cell membrane to release the viral DNA or RNA which controls the cell's metabolism to replicate itself and form new viruses. Viruses cause many diseases including influenza (single-stranded RNA), herpes (double-stranded DNA), AIDS (a RETRO-VIRUS, single-stranded RNA) and also mumps, chickenpox and polio.

viscera the organs within the body cavity, usually the abdominal cavity.

vision the capacity for sight. Light enters the EYE through the cornea and the aqueous humour. Next, it passes through the pupil, lens and vitreous humour to impinge upon the retina. There the ROD and CONE cells detect light and send impulses to the nerve fibres, impulses which are relayed to the visual cortex in the brain. *Visual acuity* is the sharpness of vision, dependent upon a healthy retina and accurate lens (*see* SNELLES CHART).

vital capacity the largest volume of air that can be exhaled after breathing in deeply.

vitamin a group of organic compounds required in very small amounts in the diet to maintain good health. Deficiencies lead to specific diseases. Vitamins are divided into two groups: vitamins A, D, E and K are fat-soluble while C and B are water soluble.

vitamin A (*or* retinol) a fat-soluble vitamin that must be in the diet as it cannot be synthesized in the body. It is essential for vision in dim light, growth and the maintenance of mucous tissue.

vitamin B a group of vitamins that, although they are not related chemically, are often found in the same types of food (*see following entries*).

vitamin B₁ (**thiamine**) active in the form thiamine pyrophosphate, a deficiency of which leads to BERI BERI.

vitamin B₂ (**riboflavin**) important in tissue respiration (enzyme reactions in cells) although a deficiency is not serious.

vitamin B₃ (**pantothenic acid**) occurs widely in foods and which is therefore unlikely to be lacking in the diet.

vitamin B₆ (**pyridoxine**) a vitamin that is important in the metabolism of several amino acids.

vitamin B₁₂ (**cyanocobalamin**) an important vitamin, in the synthesis of nucleic acids, maintenance of MYELIN surrounding nerve fibres and in the production of red blood cells. A deficiency produces anaemia and degeneration of the nervous system.

vitamin C (ascorbic acid) a vitamin essential in maintaining cell walls and connective tissue and a deficiency leads to fragility of tendons, blood vessels and skin — all characteristic of the disease called scurvy. The presence of ascorbic acid is believed to assist the uptake of iron during digestion.

vitamin D this vitamin occurs as two steroid derivations: D$_2$ or calciferol in yeast and D$_3$ or cholecalciferol which is produced by the action of sunlight on the skin. It is vital in control of blood calcium levels. It prompts an increase in calcium takeup in the gut, increasing the supply for the production of bone. It also affects phosphorus uptake. A deficiency leads to RICKETS and OSTEOMALACIA.

vitamin E a group of compounds (tocopherols) thought to prevent damage to cell membranes. A deficiency is unusual due to its widespread occurrence in foods.

vitamin H *see* BIOTIN.

vitamin K a vitamin that is essential for the clotting of blood as it is involved in the formation of prothrombin (the inactive precursor of THROMBIN) in the liver. A deficiency rarely occurs because the vitamin is synthesized by bacteria in the large intestine.

vitreous humour the jelly-like substance occurring between the lens and the retina in the EYE.

vocal cords two membranes in the LARYNX that vibrate to produce sound when air is expelled over them. Tension in the cords is controlled by muscles and tendons, thus changing the sound generated.

voluntary muscle (or striated muscle) muscle that is under conscious control, such as those muscles operating the skeleton. It consists of bundles of elongated fibres surrounded by connective tissue. A tendon at the end of the muscle attaches it to the bone. Each muscle fibre comprises smaller fibres (*myofibrils*) with alternating dark and light bands (*sarcomeres*), which produce the striated appearance and provide the contractile function.

A flexor (or *agonist*) muscle contracts becoming shorter, thus moving bones closer to each other. An extensor or *antagonist* muscle works in the opposite sense.

volvulus a twisting of part of the bowels which usually results in some obstruction which may reduce the blood supply, ending in gangrene. It may right itself spontaneously or may be righted by manipulation. However, surgery is often necessary.

vomiting (emesis) the reflex action whereby the stomach contents are expelled through the mouth, due to the contraction of the diaphragm and abdominal walls. It is due to stimulus of the appropriate centre in the brain but the primary agent is usually a sensation from the stomach itself.

vulva the external female genitals comprising two pairs of fleshy folds surrounding the vaginal opening.

vulvitis inflammation of the VULVA.

vulvovaginitis inflammation of both the VULVA and VAGINA.

W

warfarin an anticoagulant given to reduce the risk of EMBOLISM. It may be administered orally or by injection and the significant side effect is bleeding, usually from the gums and other mucous membranes.

wart (verruca) a solid, benign growth in the skin caused by a virus. There are several types: *plantar*, on the foot; *juvenile* in children and *venereal*, on the genitals. Warts are infectious and spread rapidly but will often disappear spontaneously. They can be dealt with in several ways, e.g. cryosurgery (freezing), laser treatment, and electrocautery (burning away with an electrically heated wire or needle).

water on the brain *see* HYDROCEPHALUS.

weal (or wheal) an area of the skin that is temporarily raised and coloured red, or pale with red margins. It may be due to an allergy (*see also* URTICARIA), nettle rash or a sharp blow, and in the former cases may be accompanied by itching.

webbed fingers *see* SYNDACTYLY.

Weber's test assessing a person's deafness using a tuning fork. The stem of a vibrating fork is placed on the forehead or maxillary incisors and if the hearing is normal, the sound is equal in both ears. It helps to diagnose whether hearing loss is due to a middle ear disorder or a neurosensory loss.

Weil's disease *see* LEPTOSPIROSIS.

wen *see* SEBACEOUS CYST.

Werthheim's hysterectomy a major form of hysterectomy undertaken to deal with uterine or ovarian cancer. It involves the removal of the uterus, ovaries, Fallopian tubes, upper part of the vagina and the surrounding lymph nodes.

whiplash injury damage caused by the sudden jerking backwards of the head and neck, as in a road accident. A severe whiplash can cause death, but injury is the usual outcome. The vertebrae, spinal cord, ligaments and nerves in the neck may all be damaged. Treatment usually involves wearing a special collar to immobilize the affected area.

white leg *see* THROMBOPHLEBITIS.

white matter nerve tissue in the CENTRAL NERVOUS SYSTEM, composed primarily of nerve fibres in light-coloured MYELIN sheaths. In the brain it occupies the central part of the cerebral cortex.

whitlow inflammation of tissues in the finger tip, and usually an abscess affecting the fat and fibrous tissues that comprise the pulp of the finger.

whoop the noisy and characteristic drawing in of breath following a coughing attack in WHOOPING COUGH

whooping cough (*pertussis*) an infectious disease caused by the bacterium *Bordetella pertussis*. The mucous membranes lining the air passages are affected and after a one to two week incubation period, fever, catarrh and a cough develop. The cough then becomes paroxysmal with a number of short coughs punctuated with the 'whooping' drawing in of breath. Nosebleeds and vomiting may follow a paroxysm. After about two weeks the symptoms abate but a cough may continue for some weeks. Whooping cough is not usually serious and immunization reduces the severity of an attack. However, a child may be susceptible to pneumonia and tuberculosis during the disease.

Wilm's tumour a tumour of the kidney (nephroblastoma) in infancy. Early removal of the kidney with radiotherapy and chemotherapy confers a high survival rate.

windpipe *see* TRACHEA.

wisdom tooth the last (third) molar tooth on each side of either jaw. The teeth normally erupt last, around the age of 20 to 25 although some remain impacted in the jaw bone.

withdrawal symptoms a characteristic feature when someone stops using a drug upon which they have become dependent. The hard drugs such as heroin and cocaine induce dependence as does alcohol, nicotine and amphetamines. Symptoms include shivering, tremors, vomiting and sweating.

womb *see* UTERUS.

wool sorter's disease *see* ANTHRAX.

wound a sudden break in the body tissues and/or organs caused by an external agent. There are four types based upon the result of the injury: incisions, punctures, lacerations and contusions.

wrist the joint between the hand and forearm. The wrist region comprises eight carpal bones and five metacarpal bones joined by strong ligaments. The wrist joint then articulates with the RADIUS and ULNA. The joint can move in all directions with little risk of dislocation.

wryneck (torticollis) when the head is twisted to one side due to a scar contracting or, more commonly, to excessive muscle contraction.

X

xanthelasma yellow fatty deposits in the eyelids and skin around the eyes. It often occurs in elderly people, when it is insignificant, but a severe case may be due to a fat metabolism disorder.

xanthochromia a yellow colouring, e.g. the skin in jaundice, or the cerebrospinal fluid when it contains haemoglobin breakdown products.

X chromosome the sex chromosome present in male and female although women have a pair, and men just one (with one Y CHROMOSOME). Certain disorders such as HAEMOPHILIA are carried as genes on the X chromosome.

xeroderma a condition of the skin which manifests itself as a dryness and roughness with the formation of scales. It is a mild form of ICHTHYOSIS.

xiphoid process (*or* **xiphoid cartilage**) the lowest part of the STERNUM. It is a flat cartilage that is progressively replaced by bone, a process completed sometime after middle age.

X-rays the part of the electromagnetic spectrum with waves of wavelength 10^{-12} to 10^{-9}m and frequencies of 10^{17} to 10^{21}Hz. They are produced when high velocity electrons strike a target. The rays penetrate solids to a depth that depends upon the density of the solid. X-rays of certain wavelengths will penetrate flesh but not bone. They are therefore useful in therapy and diagnosis within medicine.

Y

yawning a reflex action when the mouth is opened wide, air drawn into the lungs and slowly released. It is usually, though not exclusively, associated with tiredness or boredom.

yaws an infectious disease of the tropics caused by a spirochaete (a type of bacterium) *Treponema pertenue*, usually in unhygienic conditions. The bacteria enter through abrasions and after about two weeks, during which time there is fever, pain and itching, small tumours appear each with a yellow crust of dried serum. These may eventually form deep ulcers. The final stages may not appear until after several years and include LESIONS of skin and bone. Fortunately, penicillin works dramatically and effectively in this disease.

Y chromosome the small chromosome that carries a dominant gene conferring maleness. Normal males have 22 matched chromosome pairs and one unmatched pair comprising one X and one Y chromosome.

During sexual reproduction the mother contributes an X chromosome, but the father contributes an X or Y chromosome, XX produces a female offspring, XY male.

yellow fever an infectious viral disease in tropical Africa and South America. Transmitted by mosquitoes, it causes tissue degeneration in the liver and kidneys.

Symptoms include headache, back pains, fever, vomiting, jaundice, etc., and an attack can prove fatal. Vaccination will prove effective and anyone recovering from an attack has immunity conferred.

Z

zidovudine an antiviral drug (trade name **Retrovir**) that is used to treat AIDS. Although it slows the growth of the HIV virus, it does not effect a cure.

Zollinger-Ellison syndrome an uncommon disorder resulting in diarrhoea and multiple PEPTIC ULCERS. The cause is a pancreatic tumour or enlarged pancreas which in turn leads to high levels of the hormone gastrin which stimulates excess production of acidic gastric juice, causing the ulceration. Surgery is usually effective.

zoonosis (*plural* **zoonoses**) an infectious animal disease that can be transmitted to man. Some of the 150 or so diseases are: anthrax, brucello-sis, bovine tuberculosis, Rift Valley fever, rabies, leptospirosis and typhus (*see individual entries*).

zoophobia an unnatural and strong fear of animals.

zygomatic arch the arch of bone of either side of the face, below the eyes.

zygomatic bone a facial bone and one of a pair of bones that form the prominence of the cheeks.

zygote the cell produced by the fusion of male and female germ cells (GAM-ETES) during the early stage of fertilization, i.e. an ovum fertilized by a sperm. After passing down the FALLOPIAN TUBE, it implants in the uterus, forming the embryo.